A GUIDE TO NATURALLY BEAT HEALTH
CRISES WITH SEVEN STEPS TO RENEWAL

Our Forgotten
ALLIES

RHEA IRIS RIVERS

BALBOA.
PRESS

A DIVISION OF HAY HOUSE

Balboa Press books may be ordered through booksellers or by contacting:

Balboa Press
A Division of Hay House
1663 Liberty Drive
Bloomington, IN 47403
www.balboapress.com
1 (877) 407-4847

Because of the dynamic nature of the Internet, any web addresses or links contained in this book may have changed since publication and may no longer be valid. The views expressed in this work are solely those of the author and do not necessarily reflect the views of the publisher, and the publisher hereby disclaims any responsibility for them.

The author of this book does not dispense medical advice or prescribe the use of any technique as a form of treatment for physical, emotional, or medical problems without the advice of a physician, either directly or indirectly. The intent of the author is only to offer information of a general nature to help you in your quest for emotional and spiritual well-being. In the event you use any of the information in this book for yourself, which is your constitutional right, the author and the publisher assume no responsibility for your actions.

Any people depicted in stock imagery provided by Getty Images are models, and such images are being used for illustrative purposes only. Certain stock imagery © Getty Images.

This book is a work of non-fiction. Unless otherwise noted, the author and the publisher make no explicit guarantees as to the accuracy of the information contained in this book and in some cases, names of people and places have been altered to protect their privacy.

Print information available on the last page.

ISBN: 978-1-9822-0848-6 (sc)
ISBN: 978-1-9822-0850-9 (hc)
ISBN: 978-1-9822-0849-3 (e)

Library of Congress Control Number: 2018908307

Balboa Press rev. date: 08/02/2018

CONTENTS

ACKNOWLEDGEMENTS

I would like to express my heart-felt gratitude to the following lovelies:

Balboa Press Publishing, thank you for your patience with handling my lack of know how through the publishing experience.

Cassandra Dunn, Editor, writing is not one of my personal strengths, I can only imagine the horror you endured at the first sight of my manuscript. Thank you for your kindness and patience, it did not go unnoticed.

Veronica Cruz, Master Artist, you were able to bring a few ideas to life with your natural ability to create beauty through your artistry. You are an amazing artist, I love the cover thanks to you.

My Teachers;

Seymour Koblin, founder of School of the Healing Arts and International School of Healing Arts. Thanks to your vision many have been able to view wellness in different perspectives, with your warm, safe and loving educational environments.

John Finch, Master Herbalist, co-founder of The Self-Heal School of Herbal Studies and Healing. You were my very first teacher of herbalism and awoke my inner-healer, I am forever grateful.

Jane Richmond, Master Herbalist and Intuitive, co-founder of The Self-Heal School of Herbal Studies and Healing. Wise beyond your years, thank you for being a loving guide and bringing the ancient knowledge of our ancestors to the forefront.

Reiki Masters - Shawna Rodnunsky - Usui method Level I and II; Wendy Chaffin - Usui method Level I, II, III and Master/

Teacher; Michael Baird - Karuna Holy Fire II Master/Teacher. Thank you for the work you bring to humanity and for your loving guidance.

My son - writer extraordinaire, thank you for feeding my creative flow with your wise knowledge of the english language. Thank you for believing in me.

My daughter - thank you for believing in me and being a light in the shadows.

rheairisrivers.com
prep-4-it.com - sharing knowledge through the healing arts

PROLOGUE

In writing this book, my intention is to empower every reader with the ancient wisdom of our beautiful Mother Earth as she has everything we need to transform physical and emotional ailments. This knowledge has been forgotten by some, and is needed by all. Her energy, medicinal plants, and foods are everything and everywhere in bountiful supply, begging for our attention. The remedy for healing my own vaginal ailments, among other health crises, was found in nature, found in my kitchen, and most importantly, found within myself. Included within these pages is a 30-day guide presented as 7-Steps to Renewal. The guide is the story of how I released my body of vaginal aliments, a malignant growth and HPV in under 30 days.

To become your own healer, you need only listen to your inner-voice. One challenge in finding your solution is knowing yourself enough to sense when something feels right or wrong for you. How do certain foods, places, and people make you feel? Do you feel tired after being around certain people? Do you suffer from foggy mind after eating certain foods or drinks? The answers are within yourself, no one else can tell you these things, and they are an important part of finding your solution to self renewal. Once change has been set in motion, your daily routines shift, and so does your outcome. The beauty of change is, it is extremely reliable as it is always there, waiting for use.

This is how change can be viewed:

When we are in a health crisis, the absolute truth is that we can no longer continue with our daily rituals or routines. Our daily routine is responsible for hosting our health crisis. If we look to basic math as a step into change: if variables a + b = health crisis, then by changing the variables, you are able to find the perfect variable for the solution to your health crisis. It may very well be that one of the last variables, y + z = optimum health for you. If so, I say congratulations for digging deeper in order to know yourself and find what works for you. When we know ourselves it is pure wisdom, this wisdom can be handed down through generations, and can never be taken away from us. Change is not the enemy, change is the solution.

The journey through my health crisis is self care in its simplest form. Within this story, the technique used for seeking ancient knowledge is simple, free, and achievable. The champion through out these pages is Mother Earth (Gaia) and all of her gifts for humanity.

My intention is to share my story for all those seeking ancient healing wisdom, and to feel the interconnectedness of all beings. I cannot write about Mother Nature's healing foods and plants without discussing her energy. Energy can now be "viewed" on the SQUID Magnetometer, Taino's machines, and others. The science-minded can be assured that energy work is a true science. As a Holy Fire II Karuna/Usui Reiki Master/Teacher, I am delighted to share this fact: approximately 84% of our hospitals now have practitioners of alternative healing, including Reiki, you only need to ask for one.

My wish for you is to find all that you seek. My story defines the basis of my vaginal calamity along with other crises, and the path chose for healing. This path has been used by others with vaginal cancer, HPV, staph infection, and many other disturbances, and they too have been able to say they are free from their health crisis.

The gratitude I feel for this deep life lesson continues to grow. I now trust my inner-voice and know that, whatever the outcome, it is part of my journey. I am humbled to be a servant of Mother Earth (Gaia) and grateful for my hippie-dippie education. I share my knowledge so that I can be of service to anyone in need. In much gratitude.

To become your own healer, you need only listen to your inner-voice.

Rhea Iris Rivers, HHP
Alternative Health Consultant

Certified East / West Herbalist
Certified Nutritional Counselor
Certified Reiki Master / Teacher- Usui & Holy Fire II Karuna Reiki
Certified Classical Feng Shui Master

"So I say to you, ask and it will be given to you; search, and you will find; knock, and the door will be opened for you."

-Jesus

CHAPTER 1

What's Your Frequency

> "Knowing what you want to achieve is the first step in reaching your goal."
>
> -Unknown

In the beginning of my health crisis in 2015, I remember seeing the world through cloudy, dark eyes. It was as if I walked within my own grey cloud. I felt blah, hadn't felt amazing in years, and had grown used to it. I didn't realize what I was missing. In 2003 I began classes that opened me up to amazing new knowledge in alternative healing modalities. My main focus was to find answers to help my ADHD children make it in the world without the need of medications, and hopefully maintain their fragile self-confidence in the process. At that time, I was not aware of the depth I was being called to study. The alternative education I received was primarily for the benefit of those around me, but I can say that I too, benefited at that time.

Another mission was to find remedies for my mother's fibromyalgia, failing liver, muscular tremors, and anything to help her stop smoking. I became a research detective while trying to help those I loved, yet I felt stale and safe within the boundaries I had created for myself. At that time I was working as a hair stylist. I owned my own studio and truly enjoyed my work, as I continue to. I felt exhausted as a single parent to two great kids, while working with a clientele, and studying for nutritional counselor, herbalist and vibrational healing programs. The programs were all wonderful ways to help me feel alive, but I was depleting my core. The devastating completion of a messy, trauma-filled divorce also took its toll. Although things felt bleak, change was on the horizon.

I was also dealing with the declining health of my third child: my canine friend and best companion, Rex. He was a 14-year old shepherd mix. Rex had rescued my family 14 years prior and we all completely fell in love with him. In 2015, a few months before my diagnosis, Rex had surgery to remove a benign growth. The procedure was a success. Throughout his healing phase, I slept in his bed with him and embraced him, giving reiki energy all through those terrifying nights. When we took him to our vet's office for his check-up, the vet and his assistant said, "Most dogs this age have problems recovering from a surgery on their front leg, what are you doing?" I shared that I was doing vibrational healing with reiki, medical plants, and loving words whispered in his ear. They appeared confused.

What is your constitution?

Why do some people have physical manifestations of disease, and some seem to cruise through life unscathed? Our individual constitution has much to do with the strength of our body systems and ability to defend from disease. Our constitution is how we were formed while in the womb. Take into account what your mother put into her mouth and the quality of food and drinks consumed. What she applied topically, the quality of air, her emotional distress and her level of joy all have an effect on the strength of our core anatomy and vitality of life force. Have you noticed 80-year-olds who enjoy donuts, coffee, soda, processed foods each day, and seem to have minimal distress? My body would have given up long ago with that lifestyle!

The display of a strong constitution is due to their nourishment while in the womb, and eighty years ago genetically modified foods (GMO), sugar-laden drinks, processed food, growth hormones within our farm animals, the heavy use of pesticides, and the ascent of stress did not exist. When looking at our younger population, they appear to have more illness than previous generations, due to weaker constitutions. I would classify my core constitution as mediocre at best. As a child I was plagued with respiratory ailments and frequent bouts of strep throat, extremely painful growing pains and mono, missing weeks of school at a time. When a change in lifestyle is in motion, a weak constitution can be strengthened. Epigenetics, presented by Bruce Lipton, Ph.D., has shown less than 1% of disease is connected to genetics. When we strengthen our constitution by changing our lifestyle, poor genetics no longer dominates. (To learn more about your personal constitution, refer to the Apothecary section; under Pottengers Cats.)

Regardless of your constitution, sometimes life gets messy, and without coping skills, it can be debilitating. I lacked enthusiasm and lost myself in the abyss of spiraling thoughts and negative self-talk. My focus was in the future, and looking ahead kept me moving forward and lessened my inner turmoil, but it did not relieve stress, and it left me powerless. At the time, I didn't realize how low my own inner fire had become or how deep I was being asked to study the healing arts.

In 2015, I could see and feel lesions that felt hard and leathery, and had very thick skin around my fine china. Something was very wrong. I also noticed a gooey discharge and you know it's is bad when your fine china smells of rotting flesh, which I did not realize was me until the growth disappeared. It is said those with vaginal cancer emit the odor of a rotting corpse. Ugh. At this point, I was a Usui Reiki Master/Teacher, and was familiar with the mind-body connection to disease through our physical and emotional bodies. I understood that I was *not* feeding my body and spirit in a nourishing way, and that on some level I took part as a creator of my health crisis. But, how did I take part in its creation? What did I need to discover?

I found it a struggle to believe my somewhat healthy, alternative lifestyle could actually be behind the creation of something so potentially lethal. By changing my perspective, I was able to view hardships in my life as opportunities for growth. That is the moment I set in motion an internal dialogue of realizing my own inner-strength. I was not a victim, and the relentless indulgence of my own personal pity party had been my champion for long enough. In victim mode I thought, "Why do bad things seem to always happen to ME, why?" I came up with many reasons just to ensure that I was always correct, feeding my ego. I placed blame in every direction but my own.

When I finally shifted into owning my own creation, I set in motion the understanding that "If I am able to manifest this within myself, then I am able to heal this within myself." By changing my routines, or variables, I was able to change the outcome. With this new understanding I had to accept that what I chose to think, consume, and breathe had played an important role in creating my current health crisis. This was my catalyst to feeling more powerful than I had felt in years, and it set in motion my best detective work yet. The level of clarity was undeniable: the path I chose to live daily was not nourishing to my body, mind, or spirit and what I was doing no longer worked for me. My ego took a blow because I believed I was healthier than most people I knew. The truth was "comparison is the thief of happiness." When a lifestyle no longer nourishes its creator, its time to find a new lifestyle. In the back of my mind I had to believe this was part of my journey to wholeness, and this too would help make me stronger. I just needed a nudge.

Science defines cancer as an uncontrollable division of abnormal cells in a part of the body. Energetically, cancer can be linked to suppressing deep hurt with lifelong resentment, and possibly carrying unspoken hatred or remorse. Mentally, cancer can be linked to circular thinking about a particular subject, without decision or choice. I had hit the trifecta. I realized how many of my emotions and thoughts had been suppressed over my lifetime, and as I suffered from circulatory thinking, I realized how could I *not* have created this accumulation? When suppressed emotions dominate, it can create the perfect environment for the incubation of cancer and other disease within our physical body. The energetic body has many layers, and where a disease manifests on the physical body has an absolute correlation to where the emotional body has a blockage to the energetic flow.

In my case, the accumulation is linked to unspoken anger, keeping of deep secrets, and lack of nurturing and self-nurturing within the emotional body.

How do we shift our energetic blocks?:

When we shift our energetic frequency and raise the frequency at which we vibrate, we remove energetic blocks and move into positive life changes, including being able to manifest dreams which leave behind old patterns that no longer serve our best self. How does one go about doing this? Lifting our energetic frequency involves a conjoined effort of the physical, emotional, and mental bodies. Within this story, I share how I lifted myself to cast fine china sadness and other health crises from my being, in less than 30-days. I am an ordinary person, with an ordinary education, which happened to involve alternative healing courses. I'm sure if I could ask each reader if they have hit an unfortunate obstacle during their own life, I believe every one of us that is journeying through the chaos has came to that space where we realize this is much more difficult than we ever imagined. Somehow we found the inner strength to guide ourselves on a somewhat different path.

To begin to move our own vibrational frequency, we must talk about energy. Energy is always present, this cannot be denied. Energy can now be seen on machines, and absolutely affects our existence. Buddha has said, "Three things cannot be hidden: the sun, the moon, the truth." Energy is truth at the most basic level. It flows within, flows between, flows across, flows upside down, inside and out, can be transported, and can be stuck. Energy has everything to do with the level of frequency at which we vibrate and which health crises we host. All energy vibrates while like vibrations attract each another. When I reluctantly came to the realization that I was the creator of my health crisis, I understood the power in accountability of behavior.

Here we can see the vibrational rate in MHz at which our bodies vibrate. These ratings have been deemed accurate from Taino's Machine. This information was presented in my aromatherapy course, and I found it so interesting. I hope you find it just as interesting.

Where do you vibrate?:

Average frequency of a healthy human body	62-68 MHz
Colds and flu symptoms appear at	58 MHz
Candida at	55 MHz
Epstein Barr Virus/HPV at	52 MHz
Cancer at	42 MHz
The process of dying at	25 MHz

Cancer vibrates at 42 MHz and HPV at 52MHz, which is about where I resonated for some length of time. I was aware of my diminishing inner-fire, but couldn't piece it together.

Here is a look at how our thoughts affect our vibrational frequency:

Negative thoughts	(can lower frequency)	12 MHz
Positive thoughts	(can increase frequency)	10 MHz
Thoughts with intention	(can increase frequency)	15 MHz
(prayer & affirmations)		

Here is a look at how nutrition affects our vibrational frequency:

Processed foods	0 MHz

Whole foods – fresh, up to	15 MHz
Dry medicinal plants	12-22 MHz
Fresh medicinal plants	20-27 MHz
Coffee intake or handling, can **drop** by	12-20 MHz in 3 seconds

Pure essential oils give a range of vibrations from 52-320 MHz. The reason for this range is that when essential oils are produced, a massive amount of plant material is used. The plant material is then processed into oil, which is the strongest level of herbal preparation available.

As a certified east/west herbalist, I rarely recommend taking essential oil internally. Using an herbal tea, a whole herb, or a tincture will most always bring the body into desired health without the need for incredibly strong medicine such as an essential oil, or overuse of the plant material.

Herbology 101:

When using medicinal plant therapy, the strength of the medicine will vary depending on how the medicine was made. Depending on the length of time brewed, herbal tea (infusion) can be the mildest form of plant medicine, while also using minimal plant material. One can often feel a shift from this form of plant medicine, and it is a very effective way to receive healing.

The next level of medicinal plants is taking the whole herb, often in capsule form or as part of your diet. At this level, many can feel the body shift while using minimal plant material to achieve the desired results.

A decoction is similar to infusion, however, the plant material is boiled for a long time and left to cool for hours if need be. With this method, the plant material includes roots and barks that are too hard for infusion tea. This method is extremely medicinal, and used by ancient herbalists going back thousands of years. One would be able to feel a shift with this method of medicine. A very popular decoction is the essiac formula, which is amazing and I will discuss later in the book.

Tincture is similar to decoction, however, the medicinal plants are soaked in glycerin and/or alcohol. At this level there is most definitely a shift within a person, as tincture medicine is able to pull medicinal constituents from hard barks and roots. This form of medicine is extremely strong while using the whole herb approach and continuing to use less plant material than essential oils. To learn more about the making of these amazing methods of preparation, I recommend *The Herbal Medicine-Maker's Handbook* by James Green or *Herbal Tutor* by Anne McIntyre. These books have much of what you need to know about herbalism.

Essential oils are made through a distillation process. The type of distillation process used can affect each plant's medicinal value and vibrational frequency. Steam is most widely used, but the length of time and pressure used, as well as which batch is bottled, will affect the medicinal value (lower pressure/slower timeframe yields higher vibrational frequency and more powerful medicine). Chemical solvents or absolutes are not true essential oils (often found with rose oil) and should never be ingested due to hexane or other petrochemicals used. Carbon dioxide is a new, expensive process that produces oils under high pressure within minutes, and this process is still under investigation. Cold pressing or scarification is produced by squeezing, pressing, scraping, and shredding the outer layer of material, and is an ancient method of making essential oils.

The amount of plant material will vary depending on the plant being used in distillation.

50 pounds of eucalyptus	=	one pound of essential oil
150 pounds of lavender	=	one pound of essential oil
500 pounds of rosemary	=	one pound of essential oil
1,000 pounds of jasmine	=	one pound of essential oil
2,000 pounds of rose	=	one pound of essential oil

Now you can see why rose oil can be so expensive. The amount of material used is surprising, and shows why this medicine is precious and should be honored as such.

During the recovery phase of my health crisis, I used mostly dried and fresh herbs and tinctures internally. I used essential oil of tea tree along with other herbal allies, dried and fresh herbs, within the vaginal suppository. (The vaginal suppository formula is outlined within the apothecary section.)

Rose oil	320 MHz
Helichrysum	181 MHz
Ravensara	134 MHz
Lavender	118 MHz
Myrrh	105 MHz
Sandalwood	96 MHz
Peppermint	78 MHz
Basil	52 MHz

Essential oils that have been adulterated have a frequency of 0 MHz, which is the same with tinctures or teas that have been adulterated. When we purchase vibrational foods, herbs, or essential oils, whoever holds, moves, or touches these materials will affect the materials' vibrational frequency. When fewer people handle the solution the better the flow of energy which will yield better quality with a higher vibration solution.

A body that is high in calcium (plant calcium, sea vegetables, and algae) will have a higher vibrational frequency and be more alkaline. An alkaline body is able to heal at a much faster rate than that of an acidic body. When a body is dominated by acidity, it will have a lower frequency, and will be more susceptible to discomforts and disease.

During food preparation, I recommend using fire and exuding happiness. Fire is a living, breathing entity and has its own vibrational frequency, which is why we all enjoy a nice cook-out. The energy at a cook-out is undeniable as everyone enjoys chatting, dancing and being with one another. Fire was the catalyst for human development. When man discovered fire, man was able to make teas and herbal medicine. There is an energetic exchange during food preparation which is able to be seen, felt, and heard. Listening to beautiful music, reminding your loved ones how much they are loved, and smiling will most definitely bring up the entire room's vibrational frequency.

When choosing essential oils, medicinal herbs, and tinctures, look for wildcrafted, selected farming, and certified organic to ensure eco-farming practices for our medicinal plant community. This will ensure that integrity is one of the variables, in turn raising the vibrational frequency of Gaia and all of earth's inhabitants. Some plants are now endangered and over-harvested from the wild. When we choose products that are eco-ly crafted we give Gaia a chance to restrengthen their population:

Sandalwood and rosewood - endangered
Frankincense is close to extinction, an alternative is boswelia sacrea
Black cohosh - endangered, an alternative is baneberry
Echinacea - overly uneco-ly wildcrafted
Goldenseal, an alternative is barberry and Oregon grape
Mugwort - overly uneco-ly wildcrafted
Pipsissewa, an alternative is uva ursi and marshmallow

The term "certified therapeutic oil" is a label that is purchased and not awarded. Look for companies that have been around for decades or that can ensure the practice of eco-harvesting and quality of their batches. Consider companies which recite mantras, prayers, and play vibrational uplifting music during production to further raise the vibrational frequency.

Medicinal plants have been used for many, many years. Our great healers of the past understood the "circle of life," from nourishing tiny microbes within the topsoil and feeding our plant kingdom, to nourishing our many habitants above the topsoil. When medicinal plants are used synergistically and harmoniously, they create powerful medicine. We can utilize many parts of the plant from their roots, bark, leaves and berries to make into teas, salves, and poultices; to help return the body, mind, and spirit to vibrant health during an imbalance. Our plant allies can be used when treating bacteria which has become resistant to traditional antibiotics, successfully. When using the proper ally for an invading virus, plants are known to surround and destroy the invading virus (herpes, flu, HIV/HPV, etc,), using their very own plant intelligence. Our magnificent allies can elevate mood, detoxify organs, enhance energy or help bring sleep, without side-effects. Our forgotten allies are the silent synchronized team which require no recognition, besides caring for which they came.

"Oppression appears when we've had an experience that has shattered our view of the world, seems endless darkness, nothing lasts forever."

-Buddha

"To end suffering, embrace suffering as a part of life."

-Buddha

CHAPTER 2

Emotional Awareness

"The weak can never forgive, forgiveness is the attribute of the strong."

-Gandhi

I feel called to share my personal, somewhat embarrassing, story with you. The more honest and open I am, the more I hope this experience can help women connect with their glorious, beautiful fine china and nourish themselves in deeper, more fulfilling ways. So here it goes, I'm laying it all out. As I relay past memories, it is not my intention to belittle anyone or speak negatively, I am expressing the thoughts and emotions during the time of the memory. I feel this expression is necessary to relay the level of vibration I resonated during these times in my life. I realize sharing these experiences can be a bit of a downer, but again, I feel it necessary and hope you feel the same after reading the following chapters, when things begin to look up.

With the reality of the condition of my fine china in 2015, I was horrified, scared, sad, embarrassed, exhausted, and ungrateful.

You name it and I felt it. I had decided to keep my crisis to myself until after the holidays, so as to not bring worry to those around me. I further reduced my voice and vibrational frequency with that decision. I felt healthy in that I rarely got sick over many years. My allergies, which I had treated with Claritin for years, had also disappeared. But my core energy, my vitality, and my lust for life had gone missing. As I went through the movements of my daily routine, focused on the future, I forgot about the present. My search for more answers lead me to review past trauma in the attempt to release what maybe holding me back, stuck in lower vibrational frequency.

Memories, the seat of emotions and disease:

One of my childhood memories is of my father and mother, a time when it was their turn to go through their version of the relationship test. My father was unfaithful, as a result he and my mom separated, but not for long. I felt scared, angry and confused as a child. Since then, I've shifted my views on their relationship. My father is a good guy, and I hope you don't hate him. I came to realize that they were in a place where their relationship was unfulfilling, as many of us have also experienced. They are still married, and have been for over 50 years, and worked through whatever it was they each needed.

I've taken many lessons from this experience. I have learned compassion in maximum dosage. My father is a wonderful dad. He stood by our family and my mother daily, and cared for us, regardless of the snarls he received. He and my mother worked out what they needed in order to feel happy within their relationship. I see him now as one of the "good ol' boys," you know, the Clint Eastwood type. These guys take their lickings, stand tall when life gets rough and are always there when you need them.

My mother obviously decided to stay in the marriage. I remember I felt betrayed by her decision to stay, as if their marriage was my business. I said "I would never stay in a marriage with a cheating man" so many times growing up that I believe I created my own self-fulfilling prophecy, repeating the lesson in my own life. It wasn't until years later that I was able to see that their marital issues were their issues, and had nothing to do with me. My focus now is to love them unconditionally, to support them, and not to place judgment or ridicule.

Their relationship now is something that I could not see either of them without and brings me happiness to see them together. They have taught me about compassion and forgiveness, and what it means to stand by the ones you love. I am eternally grateful for the strength I was able to witness. Some may think this experience would reduce my vibrational frequency, and as a child I believe it did. However, now I feel full of love and admiration for the lessons this experience brought to my life, increasing my vibrational frequency in the end. I trust this experience is part of my evolution. How many layers of resentment could be connected to this memory? Have I released resentments and healed from shifting my perspective?

My next memory is unable to be retrieved fully, as I have buried it too deep. It wasn't until my realization that I was able to talk about this with friends and counselors, but my sense of knowing has remained. It is estimated that one in four girls are sexually abused in childhood from a family member or close friend. I believe the numbers are incorrect, and that it is closer to one in two girls that are sexual abused in childhood. When speaking openly with friends and clients, I have found it common to hear that they were also abused and have also buried the trauma. These are women I have known for years, and we have never shared this level of being vulnerable with each other. When one person opens up, others feel safe and share their own stories. This is before the MeToo movement, which I am happy we are finally feeling secure enough to open up, but for healing to begin all spoken memories must be factual and honest. So I ask again, "How many layers of resentment are connected to this incident in my life?" When looking within, to solve the riddle and become my own healer, I must analyze each experience that presents itself. Now is the perfect time to look within.

Again, I find lessons in compassion. My molester is dealing with his own issues. Understanding the upbringing and hardships can help to soften the pain, release the hatred, and realize that each of us are here to work on life lessons.

It saddens me to admit, but thoughts of suicide were part of my journey during the most difficult part of my divorce. I believed my children would be better off without me, due to the relentless amount of negativity and drama during what should have been their beautiful childhood. Guilt began to eat at me. My saving grace from this stream of thought was a call from my son. He called when I was deciding how to off myself as I was driving late at night. His simple and powerful words were: "What are you doing Mom?! Where are you?" As I drove aimlessly, with a tear-streaked face, I responded "I don't know. I can't do this anymore," and wept. He is very sensitive to energy, more than he realizes, and knew something was terribly wrong.

My trigger that day was a court appearance in which my ex-husband and his attorney decided not to appear. The final divorce paperwork submitted to the court had the incorrect year for our date of separation, which affected the distribution of retirement funds, another obstacle in a tower of divorce drama. This error was to be shown to the judge, so the judge could make the change on the documents. The error meant that I would lose thousands of dollars in retirement. I was experiencing an excessive amount of stress, with an ungodly amount of debt incurred from my attorney, keeping kids afloat, all while selling and moving from our home. Can you feel heaviness? Neither the ex or his attorney decided to show up for court, so I could not inform the judge of the error. It was truly a dark day.

As I look back, it's unfortunate that I placed so much value on money. Stress is one of the most debilitating forces. I had healthy, beautiful children, parents, friends, food on the table, and a roof over our heads. I had so much to be grateful for, but this incident shook me to my core, and I lost sight of any gratitude. The self-talk began again, with "How could I have ever been attracted to someone like this?" "What is wrong with me?" The victim appeared again, in what was one of the lowest points I had ever experienced, my perfect personal pity party. I reached the bottom, exhausted in the world I had created for myself, and did not trust my own decision-making. I wonder how many of us with fine china aliments and cancer have experienced thoughts of suicide? Perhaps everyone at some point thinks about what the world would be like without them, whether it would be better or worse. Do you feel thoughts of suicide would decrease our vibrational frequency, yes? By how much do you think?

After the call from my son during my late night drive, I took a look at what I must've looked like to my children. I did not like the vision I had of myself, so how could anyone else like what they saw? I was disappointed that I had allowed someone to control my thoughts and be the catalyst for depleting my self-love. I remembered being so strong in my teens and twenties. What had happened? What was I doing? Who do I want my children to see? What I realized was my life was not mine to take. I am here to learn lessons and be better than yesterday, just as we all are. We are all here to be an instrument of hope for one another, as the bigger the drama, the bigger the knowledge gained. Our gift to one another is sharing our journey, learning from one another, and living in the moment.

I fortunately received the assistance of wonderful friends to guide me through the court system during my divorce. I had released my attorney months prior, due to the insane amount of debt incurred. Standing in front of a judge, my ex-husband, and his attorney on my own was the most terrifying and gratifying experience in my entire life. I recommend this experience for anyone wanting to empower their voice. Once my ex-husband finally released his attorney, all matters were settled quickly and amicably. I believe the saying is true when retaining attorneys for divorce matters, as in our situation the drama was on overload instantly upon retaining them, and with overloaded drama comes costly attorney fees. I believe the attorneys benefit when their clients stop communicating and will throw heated coals on an already towering inferno. Without communication, there is no healing, and vibrational levels are in the negative, if there is such a thing. Of course, communication must be non-aggressive, non-finger pointing, and clear, stating only the facts, to be of real purpose.

Waiting for another court date seemed it take forever. During this period, what do you think my vibration frequency level was? I would say extremely low. Only after the ex and I were able to get in front of the judge, without attorneys, to sort out the technical terms, did I begin to feel a lift in vibrational frequency. The outcome was very uplifting. My ex decided to separate assets as of our divorce date, rather than our separation date, which was a better deal for me and I am eternally grateful. It seemed we both had learned a few of life's lessons and currently enjoy a co-parenting relationship with mutual respect at a much higher vibration.

My main lesson was to trust in the process and stop trying to control it, as we are never really in control. Release, surrender, and trust. Breathe. When things appear to be the end of the world, it is only the divine giving us another obstacle for our growth. Personally, I enjoy personal growth, and find many opportunities to grow. Therefore, the more lessons I unfold, the more feelings of gratitude I experience multiple times a day.

The late great Wayne Dyer says, "If you change the way you look at things, the things you look at change." I have found profound truth in this statement and feel my own vibration accelerate at the thought of new-found wisdom.

After I reviewed my life experiences and the manner in which I processed each memory, I could see correlations within my energy system and stuck energy within my vibrational frequency. This stuck energy invites disease physically, mentally and spiritually into our physical domain.

Let's determine where we resonate on an emotional frequency platform.

Range of Vibrational Frequency
Emotions and Feelings

How emotions can deplete vibrational frequency or how emotions can lift vibrational frequency:

Generosity - gratitude - bliss, can vibrate at the highest vibrational frequency.

Blockages of these emotions can be connected to self-destructive behavior and pineal gland calcification (metals, fluoride, and sugar toxicity will reduce our inner guidance).

Faith - love - trust, also vibrate very high and will increase your vibrational frequency. Blockages to these emotions are connected with the pituitary gland (master hormone gland) and balance of left/right sides of the brain, will affect the nervous system, nose, and ears.

Belonging - creativity - self-expression, also vibrate high. Blockages to these emotions are connected to throat, thyroid, and lung disruptions.

Compassion - passion - acceptance - self-love, also vibrate high. Blockages to these emotions are connected to heart, thymus, circulatory, and blood disruptions.

The above emotions all have an uplifting effect on one's vibrational frequency. These positive emotions release endorphins and oxytocin, they are known as the happy hormones.

* * * *

The below emotions can reduce our vibrational frequency and reduce our vitality. These negative emotions release cortisol and adrenaline, giving way to the fight or flight response, which is discussed in chapter four.

Vanity – fear - anxiety - ego: feeling these emotions can affect the physical body, stomach and digestive system, nervous system, and adrenal glands.

Betrayal - boredom - feeling the victim - lonely: feeling these emotions can affect the reproductive system (uterus, bladder, ovaries, prostate) and repress sensuality.

Dishonesty - shame - remorse - low self-confidence: feeling these emotions can affect the spinal column, intestines, penis, testicles, and fine china.

When I review the emotions I felt hostage to during the time of my diagnosis; fear, ego, betrayal, feeling the victim, and low self-confidence, I understood how my vibration was able to give way to growing my disease.

Life challenges that are brought on by vibrational-frequency-reducing emotions materialize so that we can improve and develop ourselves. When we are within a mental state of faith and trust, we transmute these emotions and ascend our vibrational frequency. These emotions are part of our growth and should (when able) be revered in highest gratitude, as their arrival has helped us become a better and more knowledgeable person. These emotions are simply part of our journey. Breathe, accept the lesson, and move forward without guilt or regret. "To end suffering, embrace suffering as a part of life." -Buddha

* * * *

The Pap Visit:
The memory of my visit with my doctor is alarming to say the least. I feel it necessary to include the discussions that transpired for

you to feel and understand where beautiful fine china resonated at that moment in time.

I arrived for my pap appointment. I scheduled the appointment as I felt something was horribly wrong with my beautiful fine china. I had small bumps and hard leathery skin along the outer rim of my labium and of course that smell. After I placed my feet in the stirrups, the doctor took one look, then excused herself to find a "colleague." As I lay there, my thoughts racing, I thought to myself, if I have an S.T.D. she would be familiar, right? I felt I had something more serious, and a surge of panic pounded through my body. The colleague entered, and my original doctor pointed to my beautiful fine china and asked, "What is that?" The colleague said, "I don't know what that is. Take a biopsy." My heart sank. If those words being spoken about your beautiful fine china wouldn't make you feel broken, what would?

A week later I received a call. I thought: this is not good, when a pap smear is normal you receive a letter in the mail as notification. I felt the pounding pressure of the adrenaline release into my system. It is terrifying how powerless the unknown can sometimes feel.

I was told that I had active HPV including many of the high-risk strains for cancer with vaginal squamous cells showing minor malignancy within the growth. The next step was to find out how deep the accumulation had grown with a colposcopy. That appointment was set for the beginning of December, which was three weeks away.

My heart pounded, anxiety raced, and I was speechless. My first thought was that I needed to find someone to blame, because I was still in a victim mindset. I thought back to during my marriage, when a routine annual pap found HPV. My body had resolved the virus out on its own. I was confused as I'd had the same partner for over 14 years, so how could this be? My OBGYN informed me HPV can lie dormant for many years without symptoms and that I could not be sure where or when I had contracted the virus. But that feeling, the knowing, was too intense to ignore.

What is HPV?

The Center for Disease Control and Prevention states, *"HPV is so common that nearly all sexually active men and women get the virus at some point in their lives. HPV is the most common transmitted virus in the U.S."* It is estimated over 70% of Americans are infected, while numbers increase 14% annually. There are over 100 different strains of HPV while at least 13 are cancer-causing or high risk. When looking to our forgotten allies for nourishing answers, Gaia has gifted humanity with many antiviral plants. The *virus is just a virus* and in the medicinal plant world it does not matter which strain you host, plant intelligence is part of the solution: dosage, how frequently and how much to consume is most important. The dosage while in healing crisis should be every 1 to 3 hours, to allow movement of stuck physical blockages to shift.

We have many antivirals to chose from. The top seven antiviral herbs as listed by Stephen Harrod Buhner, author of Herbal Antivirals are: *Chinese skullcap, elder, houttuynia, isatis, licorice, lomatium, and ginger.* One of my favorites is *poke root*, which has been shown to relieve mice of an HIV infection and will be highlighted throughout the book. Poke root is also part of my vaginal suppository formula, as discussed within the Apothecary. *Neem* Oil is another favorite, and has been known to defeat the herpes virus, is a great intercourse oil as it will kill sperm and keep viral and bacterial infestations away (soak an organic cotton ball, insert into fine china for 15 minutes, remove before intercourse). *Neem* leaf is effective at preventing the development of malaria and is *toxic to antibiotic resistant strains of malaria.* The oil is used as insect repellent topically for mosquitos, biting flies, sand fleas and ticks. It is also used in organic farming practices to keep pesky bugs away while not harming our nectar-loving flying beauties. These are only a few of the job duties these amazing allies are responsible for.

Who to blame?:

As I think back to my first diagnosis, during that time in my life, my ex traveled a lot for work, which I believed was good for a certain length of time. But I suspected he was being unfaithful, as we were both unfulfilled. If I had been the one traveling around for my job, free as a bird, I'm not sure what I may have done. We had grown in opposite directions, so that I felt like a stranger was with me most of the time. I felt stuck, and that immoveable stuck energy showed itself in other ways. At the age of 40 I blew out my knee playing court volleyball, and then the same happened to my other knee at 42. The energetic connection to a knee injury is the inability to make a decision and move forward in life, and the inflexibility of thought patterns when denying the heart as the guide. Basically, I was on the wrong bus, with my body going one way, and my spirit going the other. My body was trying to tell me, giving hints or whispers, but I am hard of hearing at times. By choosing to leave the marriage I would like to believe that I showed my daughter you can overcome any obstacle in life, to listen to all sides with an open heart, and to never become the doormat. For my son, I would like to believe I showed him to never take things for granted, to listen to all sides before making decisions and to value all opinions different from his own. Essentially, I hope both learned compassion and heartfelt open communication to break the unhealthy cycle both my ex and I allowed them to witness.

What I found most unforgivable about being unfaithful, was bringing in other partners and choosing not to wear protection while with other people. On some level that felt like more of a betrayal than the actual betrayal. I buried most of those feelings, as when I brought up the subject I was judged as jealous. Therefore, healing was unable to transpire within the relationship. Also, the first man I dated after my separation was too unfaithful. We dated for over a year and were both tested for STDs before we removed our protection. There is *not an HPV test for men,* and they rarely have symptoms. Regardless, it turns out he was also unfaithful, and also chose not to wear protection, as it was revealed after I confronted him and her. Do you feel a connection to my attraction to men who are unable to be loyal? Have I been recreating my childhood trauma in order to work through it? What was I viewing in the wrong perspective? How much of this memory attributes to my depleting vibrational frequency?

Looking back in our past is part of knowing where we need work in the present, but spending too much time in the past will cause disempowerment in the present. I found myself wanting to find someone to blame, which you can see from the previous paragraphs. I found myself slipping into victim mode once again, obsessively reviewing the past. The present tense is the only tense where we can heal ourselves and be fully empowered. I have studied this time and time again, and yet old patterns can still emerge.

But this time I was ready to be the observer of these thoughts after my diagnosis, and not the performer. I was grateful for the meditation and communication courses I attended, and they will be highlighted throughout this book. I released thoughts of being the victim, as it was not for the best and highest interest of myself. It didn't matter where I had contracted the virus, I had it and supplied the perfect environment and nourishment for its growth. *I was responsible. Solely. Irrevocably.* To add to the lesson, each of these relationships displayed red flags. I did not honor my inner-knowing or trust in the process.

Finding inner-guidance:

The technique I used to find my inner-guidance was taught during a course from Doreen Virtue called Assertiveness Communication, which is reviewed in depth in chapter five. It is simple, effective, and able to be used any time, any place. To become empowered within the present moment, we must know where we stand on issues and how we feel. What can be better than slowing down and checking in with yourself?

Next step was to determine the source of my fear in sharing my diagnosis:

Simply close your eyes as you sit comfortably, and inhale deeply, then open-mouth exhale a few times, and then breathe normally. Within each breath, release more and more stored tension. Relax your face, shoulders, arms, lips, belly, legs, and breathe. *It is believed that in the breath we receive messages from our higher self, our inner-fire for inspiration and heavenly guidance.* In fact, on every continent there is evidence of meditations or prayers beginning with breath work. **When we _pray_, we _speak_ with the divine, and when we _meditate_, we _listen_ to the response of the divine.** Once relaxed, mentally follow the emotion back to its origin.

I was finding the source of my fear around sharing my diagnosis. I relaxed and asked myself (called body scanning): is my fear caused from telling my parents about my health? I envisioned the interaction and checked in with how it made me feel. I concluded that telling my parents was not the origin of my fear. I did the same for friends and concluded that was not the origin of my fear. Then, I envisioned telling my children, and had a feeling of heightened heartbeat, fear and tightness in my throat. I concluded this was the origin of my fear.

To release fear, it is best to come clean. Address the person(s) with your concerns. Speak directly from an "I feel" stance, without accusations, and take full responsibility. (For example: "I feel anxious about sharing this information with you, and causing you worry." Or "I feel I may lose your support if I share this information, so please know I value you being a part of my life.") I informed my children of my diagnosis on our car ride up to visit their grandparents for Thanksgiving. I felt that driving could be a distraction and might make it easier for all of us. Upon spilling the beans, I felt a complete shift in the level of our happiness and how we connected and supported one another. My wonderful daughter held my hand and whispered sweet love my way, and I will never forget her healing touch, tears, and words of love. My wonderful son about jumped from his skin, and held me from the back seat. His words of wisdom never cease to amaze me. He said, "Mom, you have been studying this stuff for years. This is your thing! You can do this." His words caught me off guard. Talk about a moment of clarity, wow. He was completely correct. I just did not believe in myself the way he believed in me and had not realized so. Would having the support of those you love increase or decrease your vibrational frequency? Absolutely increase. I felt my inner fire begin to ignite.

In my mind, I envisioned them being disappointed in me and dis-valuing my alternative healing education, closing themselves off to alternative healing for their entire lives. Ugh! No wonder I had fear. They felt comforted and confident in my education and this gave me the inner fire I needed and longed for. I rarely had felt supported for my alternative education. Most of my marriage community had been closed to anything alternative. This was the early 2000s to 2010, and people were just beginning to awaken to natural healing. I was ahead of the pack.

Source of passion for the healing arts:

The only reason I was ahead of the pack was because of my catalyst: keeping my children off ADHD medication. It just felt wrong. Back then I was already checking in with how choices affected my well-being by body-scanning. Why would I medicate these beautiful, healthy children just to slow them down? There had to be another way. I realize as I write these words that I am better about hearing my inner-voice when it concerns others than I am when it concerns myself.

At what age do our children become the teacher? Oh, yes, at birth. To be a parent is the most selfless act of unconditional love, in my opinion. I chose to take my family on its own path, step up my parenting techniques, and study all I could about healing ADHD naturally with reiki, nutrition, communication, herbs, and feng shui. My children needed smaller classroom sizes and positive reinforcement, which meant taking them out of the public school system. I left no stone unturned as I looked for answers for my family, as many mothers have done before me. We are the perfect detectives when family love is involved.

What I found was much more than I dreamed of: a new path in life which has become more fulfilling than I could have imagined. Our overactive children are our leaders, as they are not afraid to question authority or do things in an entirely new way. If they do not hold their teacher in high regard, they will simply tune out and create their own new way of holding class, usually focused upon themselves. They are highly intuitive and frequently cannot differentiate between the chaotic energy around them or identifying the energy as their own. These sensitive children are our gifts and most are unfortunately medicated to slow them down in an attempt to make them fit in with the rest of society. Rarely in history do our leaders fit in anywhere, it is the rest of society that changes to fit in with them. Let's take a moment to look at the state of our current leaders. Most of us wonder why we seem to never have better choices during elections. I believe our true leaders have all been snuffed out from childhood trauma. I'm not saying my children will rule the world one day, but at least whatever they choose to become, they will be able to have multiple tools to use by way of knowing themselves, for any journey they choose.

Would spilling the beans, being comforted, loved, and encouraged, raise or reduce my vibrational frequency? My frequency raised the roof and I was on a roll. I felt these obstacles has been put in front of me so that I could learn more of self love.

"Fear is an illusion, it does not exist, it is created in the mind."

-Miguel Ruiz

CHAPTER 3

Nutritional Guidance

"We can never obtain peace in our outer world until we make peace with ourselves."

-Dalai Lama

With an alternative view, I no longer felt like a powerless victim, whining and placing blame. I felt empowered to become my own rescuer, my own healer. If others could defeat horrible disease naturally, then why couldn't I also defeat disease naturally? Likewise, if I am able to defeat disease naturally, then why couldn't others do the same? My wish is for each reader to find their catalyst and grow to their heart's desire.

After the diagnosis, I had a few weeks before the colposcopy. I believed I was in the perfect place at the perfect time. I was working on feeling grateful to be able to use my ancient alternative knowledge. My intention was to have a clear colposcopy and kick this disease the hell out of me. Time was short and I had much work to do.

During this part of my research, I focused on the energetic connection to cancer and why it chooses to grow in certain parts of the body and at a particular time in life. What I discovered opened up new layers of understanding disease and how cancer grows. In the case of vaginal cancer, the uterus and vaginal walls store years of resentment, sexual trauma, and/or unspoken emotions. This beautiful body part acts as its own entity or micro-eco system. This trauma is stored in the lining of the uterus, like a chipmunk would store acorns for a long winter. This amazing organ is very sensitive and needs to be nourished with love, open communication, honesty, and most importantly, good ol' clean fun. The wounds of past sexual abuse, putting others before self care, and never opening up with assertive heartfelt communication are major contributors in vaginal health. Would a constant suppression of releasing matters of the heart reduce our vibrational frequency? Yes, it would squash it. Much of this research was with the beautiful Louise Hay, founder of Hay House and a fellow kick the shit out of vaginal cancer girl.

I continued my research into healing and what I found next continues to make me smile. The irony. Prior to my diagnosis, for seven-eight months or so, my glorious fine china was not being shined or buffed. What I am saying is that I was getting zero action, no sex, a complete shut-down. The shut-down was linked to emotional distress, poor nourishing foods and lack of vitality. When the physical body creates a barrier like accumulations of squamous cells, the road to recovery is rooted deeply within the emotional body. The fine china is good at creating barriers, i.e., chronic yeast infections, bacterial infections, candida overgrowth, hormone disruptions, endometriosis, cysts, cancer, etc. These barriers are an invitation to evaluate your lifestyle. They are signals from the physical body stating: "I'm not happy here." You can ask yourself if your partner needs to cleanse his/her own level of bacteria or candida. Is your partner reinfecting you? Is your partner communicating on a level to excite fine china? Are you communicating on a level to nourish fine china? Do you have too many partners? Does your partner have other partners? Does your toy need a good scrub down? Are you consuming nourishing foods and liquids? There are so many variables. Simply check-in with yourself.

The irony was I believed taking a break in relationships and intercourse would be great to give myself a rest, which was emotionally beneficial. However, intercourse is actually very good for glorious fine china. The energy and blood flow to and around glorious fine china acts as a filter. The energy and blood flow allows for an exchange emotionally, energetically and physically. This removes old stagnant energies, and makes way for new energy to occupy the area. So then, one is able to move on with good ol' clean fun. (Please do not become promiscuous on my account, I believe one wonderful partner is exactly what we need.)

Nourishing Diets:

A few months before my diagnosis, I attended a comparative nutrition course with research papers due on each diet presented. I enjoyed learning so many ancient diets but felt overwhelmed. After getting off work, I would go through a drive-through and pick up Mexican food (a bean tostado to be exact) as well as other processed foods. I realized this was not a health food -with the GMO corn tortilla, whatever is in bean's lard, Crisco, yellow cheese- but I drove my car through, placed the order and handed over my money. This allowed me the time to complete my studies, and got me off my tired feet. At the time, I said to myself "When I've completed this course, I will take time to meal prep."

During my comparative nutrition course, I felt the need to find the "best" diet and compared each course relentlessly. I studied Ayurvedic nutrition, whole foods nutrition, clinical nutrition, macrobiotics, and raw foods. What I discovered is that each diet is great for the right person. It is up to the individual to look within and feel which is best for oneself. These five nutritional lifestyles are the basis of all diets. My position as an alternative health consultant is to guide an individual into their best version, not to dictate, ridicule or control them. For my best self, I find raw foods (mostly juices and smoothies) and macrobiotics the perfect match to my anatomy.

Let's review the main purpose of food. Food is simply used by the body to nourish and bring energy to our different body systems. Therefore, the main purpose of meal time is not to bring pleasure to the senses; well at least not every meal (noted as gluttony). When we fall into the rut of continuously pleasing the senses we tune out the information given from our inner-guidance, whispering which nourishing foods our anatomy needs. By over-eating or craving foods and drinks that bring pleasure to the senses, we become host to a low vibrational frequency. Foods such as ice cream, cookies, chocolate, chips, hot dogs, cocktails, wine, coffee, etc. These foods belong on the "dessert tray." The dessert tray is consumed once in a while, or *not ever* consumed while in a healing crisis. Fun fact: desserts spelled backwards is stressed. Cookies would be my pleasure to the senses.

Pleasure foods can and will become addictive to the physical and emotional bodies. The mind will give you every reason why you *should* continue with your addiction. Things like: I only consume this one time a day and it is the only food I truly love - or - I gave up this one addiction and this other addiction is all that I have left. Sound familiar? But once you have cleared the addiction cycle from your lifestyle the desire to consume or over eat will reduce dramatically. To bring awareness to the addiction is the first step in changing the lifestyle pattern, by checking in with yourself.

Let's look at treating these addictions energetically: if you crave sweetness, bring more self-nurturing into your lifestyle. Tell someone how much you enjoy their company, love unconditionally, and treat yourself to a bath. If you crave spicy fried foods, try to bring more variety into your life. Go out dancing, attend a rock concert, and laugh until your stomach aches. *There is an energetic connection to the amount of food we crave, which foods we crave and the emotional emptiness we are attempting to fill.*

If you are one to continuously over eat, and then find yourself wondering: why do I consume foods in such large quantities? Now is a good time to search within yourself to uncover what is missing from your life. To fill an emotional void, you can open yourself to new experiences, i.e., become a foster parent for our fur babies and/ or our human babies, or volunteer a few hours spending time in our senior retirement communities with lonely souls. When we fill the emotional body we then feed the physical body, reducing health crises and unhealthy cravings. Be open during your body scan to release un-nurturing relationships, change employment, or move your physical residence, if you are being guided to do so.

I believe most people are aware of GMO foods, but just in case, corn production within the United States is almost all genetically modified: 88% of the entire crop. The largest GMO crops are wheat, corn, and soy, but they do not stop there. GMO food is linked to hormone disorders, auto immune disorders, and gut bacteria imbalance. GMO farming practices also have many drawbacks, such as leaching the nutrients from the soil after continuously replanting the same crop. Also, with GMO seeds used in American farming the use of glyphosate, a chemical found in Roundup herbicide, is linked to carcinogenic activity and is lethal to human cells. GMO seeds, "fake seeds," have been designed to survive the heavy application of herbicides like glyphosate and increase the toxic load of our food supply. Of course one of the most important drawbacks is the depletion of the earth's top soil. The beneficial microbes living within the soil are destroyed as well as our beautiful flying pollinators. With the demise of our topsoil and our natural pollinators how are we to feed and nurture our children or our children's children, and so on. When I became a conscious consumer I felt the need to nourish not only my own body but all of humanity and our beautiful planet earth. Our most powerful use of our voice is how we choose to spend our money.

Many of these disruptions have been linked to vaginal cancer. (A wonderful book on the condition of our food supply and the condition of our topsoil is *Planet Heal Thyself* by Jordan Rubin. This book is full of ancient wisdom and Jordan states the facts wonderfully.) I had created the perfect incubator for the disease with the activation of HPV, high levels of stress, poor nutritional intake, and a low level of vibration. When you own and understand the power of your own behavior, you can then change that behavior to achieve the desired results.

Healing diet during my health crisis:

During my healing phase, my diet was a blend of macrobiotics and raw foods. I prepared each of my own meals. When you dine out, please know all items on the menu will be genetically modified and low vibration unless the menu states otherwise. Believe me, the restaurant will definitely be shouting about the fact they are non-GMO and organic if that is the case. While in healing crisis your meals should be made at home in your kitchen otherwise known as your medicine cabinet.

Macrobiotic means "big life." George Ohsawa is the founder of this miraculous diet. This man cured himself of tuberculosis at the age of nineteen. He witnessed his entire family pass from this horrible disease, and was able to see that his family's lifestyle was a big part of their ill health. He decided to try something different, and to view the situation with a new perspective. He saved his own life and many others with this amazing new approach to food. Macrobiotics is the balance of yin (expanding) and yang (contracting) energies. There are too many variables to go through them all within this book. I recommend further study with an additional book, referenced at the end of the chapter. In the most basic form, use food that is currently in season, and envision your kitchen as your medicine cabinet.

Many people have changed their perspectives in order to change an outcome. This concept is nothing new. It is ancient knowledge being recycled. Wayne Dyer said, "When we change the way we look at things, the things we look at change." This is one of my favorites quotes of all time, that is why I had to use it twice.

Every one of my meals was energized with reiki, I chewed each mouthful thirty times, and I gave gratitude to Gaia, or whatever calls you, for another great meal. All of which have an uplifting effect on vibrational frequency.

Breakfast

I started my day with raw juice and/or grain porridge. I used apple juice, cinnamon, maple syrup, and dates as natural sweeteners, but only one at a time and very little. (*Porridge received its name long ago, when "the poor" consumed mostly grains. The nobles' diet was based on animal products such as milk, eggs, cheese, meat, and wine. The "poor" commoners noticed that diseases like diabetes, gout, and heart disease were seen with the nobles, but not the "poor" commoners. The commoners may have died form starvation or other issues, but not the diseases of the nobles.*)

My morning porridge was of oats, quinoa, spelt, and amaranth. I added nuts, sprouts, berries, and organic coconut oil or olive oil.

I kept fruit and sweeteners to a minimum, as *all sugar will grow cancer*, even fructose. My raw juice was mostly vegetables (kale, avocado, carrot, celery, beet, dandelion, watercress, cucumber, spinach, burdock, parsley, cilantro, lime, lemon, basil, and spirulina) with some pineapple, berries, or apple for taste. I also added sprouts, ginger, garlic, chia seeds, cacao, cinnamon, and/or cayenne pepper. I made a blend of these ingredients and didn't use every ingredient at one time. I scanned my body daily and asked what I wanted each day or found fun recipes online, allowing my love for food prep to climax.

The important part of bringing raw foods into your diet is that raw foods are active, living food, full of vibrational frequency. Raw food is full of beneficial enzymes, and can clarify, heal, and cleanse the entire body, mind and spirit. Raw food has an alkalizing effect that is exceptional at feeding collagen production and maintaining youthfulness. For cellular regeneration, it is recommended to remain on raw foods for four months, to allow the body time to heal itself as well, as the body takes 120-days to replenish with new fluids. Currently, raw morning juice is part of my routine, this allows the digestion to rest and relax. However, I do not believe a diet of entirely 100% raw food is beneficial long term. The hard, raw foods (cruciferous and root vegetables) can lie in the gut and are too hard to be digested effectively or continuously. These foods will ferment in the gut to a toxic state, producing harmful gases and causing harm to the beneficial flora. (When mankind discovered fire, we evolved from the Neanderthal mind and were then able to prepare medicine and prepare meals.) My diet was in moderation with a variety of foods. The more variety within our lifestyle the more nutrients we are able to give our bodies.

Chlorella and cilantro can eliminate 87% of lead toxins, 91% of mercury, 74% of aluminum, and are essential in clearing pathways within the pineal gland-raising vibrational frequency and allow for inner-guidance to be heard.

Lunch and Dinner

I usually made a large morning juice and sipped it through lunch time. I would prepare a grain, vegetable and leafy green concoction. I soaked and sprouted all of my grains and legumes. This is a macrobiotic recommendation and is highly nutritive for our entire being. Research has shown civilizations with the highest levels of consciousness chose a diet rich in grains and vegetables, i.e., Egyptians and Mayans. Back then grains were obviously non-GMO, with zero pesticides / herbicides, grown with vibrant clean water. They were soaked, touched, and cooked lovingly, in full gratitude, and practically worshipped. All of which makes a difference in how the body utilizes the grain, including spiritual development. I prepared, soaked, or sprouted grains and legumes daily, and sautéed them with vegetables for delicious stir fries. For the perfect protein, mix rice and beans, and you can also use other sea vegetables (kombu, dulse, wakame) for maximum nutritional intake. At the end of the Apothecary is a soaking and sprouting guide.

I would begin the soak the day before my day off, then prepare a pot of grains and a pot of legumes (beans) for the entire week on my day off. I'd store them in the refrigerator, then add them to whatever I was making each day. My go-to grain is brown rice, barley, and millet, and for legumes I like a variety of adzuki, pinto, lentil, and kidney beans. Just choose one and begin, and you will figure out your favorite.

Miso

I consumed this special soup a few times a week. Miso is fermented soy, which means it is very high in good bacteria and enzymes, and contains an abundance of vitamins, proteins, and minerals. Miso will alkalize the blood and is also great for someone going through chemo or radiation. Miso will minimize radiation effects on the body. *Research has shown that those who consumed wakame (sea vegetable) with miso soup daily had minimal toxins from the horrific events at Hiroshima.* Miso has also been found to repress the growth of cancerous tumors. The older the miso, the more beneficial the bacteria levels. Aged and fermented soy must be non-GMO. *Miso becomes an anti-estrogenic food when pure.* Genetically modified soy has none of these health benefits. My miso soup was mixed with prepared grains and/or legumes, shiitake mushrooms, bok choy, seaweed (wakame, kombu, or nori), carrot, celery, peppers, daikon radish, onion, a dash of shoyu or soy sauce, and a dash of sea salt. I focused on what was in season and looked welcoming. Miso should never be boiled. Boiling miso will kill the beneficial flora.

Other fermented foods I consumed were sauerkraut, kimchi, and pickled vegetables.

I made my own dressings and topped grain salads and green salads with miso, lemon, garlic, olive oil, ginger, different vinegars, and garden herbs. I just got creative, using whatever sounded good. My favorite dressing is simple: olive oil, balsamic vinegar, and lemon with a touch of maple syrup or honey. These dressings will stay fresh for a week or so in the refrigerator. Enjoy.

Warm Drinks

Green tea with dandelion tincture, daily. I infused the green tea for just a few minutes.

The pesky weed, dandelion, is highly nutritive, with cal/mag and vitamin K. Its leaves are great in salads or juiced, and can balance blood sugar, balance hormones, work as a liver tonic for detoxification, and can clear skin.

Golden tea with homemade almond milk or coconut milk or fresh coconut water, turmeric, fresh ginger, clove, cinnamon, nutmeg, cardamom, cayenne pepper, lemon, and sometimes mixed with cacao. I enjoyed this drink and still do, regularly.

Sweet vegetable drink with equal amounts of onion, carrot, cabbage, and sweet winter squash, finely chopped. Add to 4x amount of water, cover, boil on low for 20 minutes, then strain and drink the liquid, saving the vegetables for stir-fry or soup. This stabilizes blood sugar, softens the pancreas, relaxes the body and muscles, and is delicious.

Multiple herbal teas, such as chamomile, licorice, astragalus root, rose, ginger (fresh), rose hips, red raspberry leaf, peppermint, nettles, holy basil, whichever sounded best, or sometimes I would create my own brew by combining different herbs.

Water Source

I consumed water that was filtered of fluoride, and was chlorine-free and additive-free, as these will destroy the gut flora, and what do we know? All disease is rooted in the gut. Never use ice or cold water, this will slow the energetic movement of the body systems, reducing vibrational frequency. Fresh coconut water straight from the coconut was also consumed and been shown to destroy cancer cells.

Baths

Hot Himalayan salt/epsom baths with different herbs in the water were also part of my healing phase.

I took a cold rinse after the bath to activate circulation, strengthen immunity, and keep my hair, skin, and nails looking beautiful.

Skin Brushing

With a bamboo brush, stroke toward the heart to reduce toxicity and activate the circulatory system. This helps to discharge fat deposits and release toxins. Doing this before or after the bath, not during, is best.

Tongue Scraping

Literally pulling from the deep part of the throat. 70% of toxins are released on the breath, 20% of release is from the skin, 7% is from urination, and 3% is from bowel release.

Oil Pulling

Use organic coconut oil or bentonite clay liquid to pull toxins from the teeth and gums. Hold the liquid for 10 to 20 minutes in your mouth, then spit it out in the garbage.

Cooking

I cooked all grains and legumes thoroughly.

I kept the heat low while preparing soups and stir-fries, as low heat preserves the living vibration and enzyme activity of the vegetables.

Never use corn oil. Corn, wheat, and soy are the highest GMO foods.

Capsule Herbs

Herbal Medicinal Allies in whole capsule form were taken frequently and will be outlined under the Apothecary section; Herbal Ally Capsules.

Suppositories

Herbal Medicinal Allies were made into super powerhouse suppositories and will be outlined under the Apothecary section; Fine China Suppository.

Just keep it simple. Get to know your kitchen. Play uplifting music. Let your friends and family know how much you love to cook for them. Visit local farmer's markets and see what is growing around you. Hand select. Variety is the spice of life, so mix it up.

* * * *

Removing foods from your diet is just as important as what you decide to bring into your diet. I avoided these foods and actions during my healing phase:

OMIT:
All meat
Soda
Dairy
Sugar
Anything baked with flour
Pasta
All packaged foods

I limited foods with estrogen: tofu, flax, sunflower seeds, sunflower oil, except for miso, which has an anti-estrogen effect on the body

Anything pasteurized, as after pasteurization food becomes processed and loses all of its vibration, and is then dead food

Powered protein: isolated protein has adverse effects on our health, (the truth about protein powder is at the end of this chapter)—it is a processed dead food

Cooking with electricity, as this method gives zero in vibrational frequency

Coffee: caffeine pulls energy from the adrenals, from our own resources, and reduces the vibrational frequency (the truth about coffee is at the end of the chapter)

Alcohol is toxic for the body systems, turns to sugar, and makes it difficult to tune into what is best for oneself

Frozen foods or chilled drinks: ingesting cold foods slows the digestive process and in turn will slow the flow of energy, reducing the vibrational frequency

All fragrance and perfume (can cause hormonal imbalance), chemical deodorants or antiperspirants (it is unnatural to not perspire, and chemicals increase toxicity levels) I used neem oil or coconut oil mixed with lemon

Beauty products made with chemicals. My favorites; Miessence, Lenus, and Simply Divine Botanicals are truly remarkable, high vibrational clean products

Chemical-laden sanitary pads. I used organic cotton and ceased all tampon insertion

Toilet paper with fragrance, bleach or chlorine

Chemical-laden condoms. Use organic condoms, purchase your own - do not expect someone else to buy the best for your fine china

Why Soak? Whole Grains, Nuts, Seeds:

Always NON-GMO and Organic.

Why would we choose to soak or sprout? One of many reasons is to increase the absorption of polyphenols, an essential antioxidant. The outer husk of the grain contains enzyme inhibitors, and without soaking, the inhibitors can cause digestive disturbances. These inhibitors prevent adequate digestion, absorption of vital nutrients, and can cause allergic reactions in some people, i.e. IBS, colitis, GI tract inflammation.

By sprouting or soaking, nutrients including amino acids (the building blocks of proteins), copper, iron, zinc, vitamin B1, magnesium, and enzymes become more available and easier to absorb. For example, studies have found that folate increases in sprouted grains up to 3.8 times, and show increases in vitamin C and E, beta-carotene, proteins, and antioxidants, with peak concentrations of nutrients observed after 5 days of sprouting.

With soaking or sprouting, food becomes easier to digest, decreases inhibitors and phytic acid, increases protein availability, increases fiber content, breaks down gluten for easy digestion, helps reduce other allergens found in grains, and increases enzymes and antioxidants.

This is ancient cooking, the way our great grandmothers knew. How to soak and sprout is found at the end of the Apothecary.

Health Issues Associated with Coffee and Caffeine:

One of the main health issues in today's world is exhausted adrenal glands and endocrine system malfunction. While you enjoy the buzz off a cup of morning java, you imagine the caffeine soaring through your veins and revitalizing your senses. But this is misleading. Our body is not getting buzzed off the caffeine, our adrenal glands are secreting adrenaline and cortisol, the hormones your body depends on in emergencies to elevate your heart rate, increase your respiration and blood pressure, giving way to the fight-or-flight response. When you overuse this stimulant, the adrenals become exhausted. If you have 1, 2. or 3 cups of coffee daily and still sleep at night, guess what? Your adrenals have completely given up responding. This means you have less resistance to stress, which leaves you vulnerable to health hazards such as environmental pollutants and disease. Take into account the level of our personal constitution which each person has a varying beginning point.

As we age, the adrenals become more and more important to maintain vitality. They are the production center of essential youth and sex hormones, including DHEA progesterone, testosterone, and estrogen. Many people find as they age that they can no longer tolerate the same level of caffeine consumption as in their earlier years.

The adrenals are considered the storage center for your vital force: your reservoir of energy. They need nourishing to keep them in optimal health. Think of your adrenals as your 401K account. If you continue to make withdrawals without any nourishing deposits, you will hit rock bottom with a deficit in the form of depleted vitality and health.

Sever Blood Sugar Swings - Caffeine forces the liver to release glycogen into the blood stream. The pancreas responds to the sudden rise in blood sugar by releasing insulin, the hormone which causes excess carbs to be stored as fat. A sharp blood sugar drop results in a state of hypoglycemia. That is when you think you need another cup of java and the cycle repeats.

By achieving hormone balance and blood sugar stability, you can maintain your natural weight and optimal energy level. The breakdown of caffeine causes the pancreas to release too much insulin, thus creating a climate in which excess carbs are stored as fat and are unavailable for use as energy by your brain. Although caffeine is a metabolic stimulant, the ultimate effect is to increase your appetite and contribute to weight gain, therefore caffeine should be avoided by anyone working to reduce body fat.

Acid Imbalance - Coffee hosts over 208 acids, and can contribute to indigestion and a wide variety of health problems resulting from over-acidity. This has been associated with arthritis, rheumatic issues, skin irritations, and digestion complaints such as colitis and IBS. Many people experience a burning sensation in their stomach after drinking coffee because coffee increases the secretion of acid in the stomach. Optimal vitality calls for an alkaline pH balance in the body.

Essential Mineral Depletion - Coffee inhibits the absorption of some nutrients and causes the urinary excretion of calcium, magnesium, potassium, iron, and trace minerals, which are all essential elements necessary for good health. Women should be concerned about osteoporosis as menopause sets in. Studies show that women who drink coffee have an increased incidence of osteoporosis compared to non-coffee drinkers. Men are not immune to osteoporosis, either.

The are a number of health conditions linked with the over-consumption of coffee.

Acid indigestion	Anxiety, irritability, nervousness
Candida and yeast problems	Colitis, diverticulitis, diarrhea
Irritable bowel symptoms	Chronic Fatigue Syndrome
Autoimmune disorders	Diabetes or hypoglycemia
Heart disease	High blood pressure
Insomnia and interrupted sleep	Liver disease
Gallbladder problems	Gallbladder stones
Kidney problems	Kidney stones
Migraines and headaches	Osteoporosis
Skin irritations, rashes, dryness	Ulcers, heartburn, hiatal hernia
Urinary tract irritation	Hormone disruption

Female Health Issues - Women need to be concerned about their caffeine intake during pregnancy, because caffeine crosses the placental barrier to the fetus. Studies show caffeine consumption is linked to a higher incidence of miscarriage, infertility, and low birth weight. PMS symptoms and fibrocystic breast disease are both aggravated by caffeine. Hot flashes caused by hormonal fluctuations during menopause also are aggravated by caffeine. Coffee causes the body to excrete calcium and other minerals. Women at risk for osteoporosis should eliminate coffee and caffeine.

Male Health Issues - Coffee is an irritant to the urinary tract and bladder. It is also a diuretic that aggravates conditions associated with frequent urination. Eliminating coffee and caffeine relieves symptoms associated with frequent urination due to enlarged prostate glands.

Information obtained from:

INTERNATIONAL COLLEGE OF HOLISTIC STUDIES
INTERNATIONAL SCHOOL OF HEALING ARTS
JEREMY E. KASLOW MD, FACP, FACAA
    Health issues associated with coffee and caffeine
THE ZONE by BARRY SEARS

Truth About Isolated Protein and Protein Supplements:

Protein supplements can be used as a wonderful tool for change, to help to promote muscle growth. But they can also be the cause of many health issues. Short-term protein supplements can be used in weigh-loss programs, and some have amazing results. But as we age we shift, and with long-term use, we begin to see negative side effects.

Protein supplements are processed, which means they lack the vital vibrational energy essential for our body to maintain optimum health. The protein is taken out of its original source and made into an isolated compound, which can then be trademarked and sold at elevated costs for consumption. Also, the amount of protein is too much for the body to utilize because it is simply unnatural.

What does that mean? Nature has shown us that when we separate components of plants, we are sure to see negative side effects prevalent in the body. We cannot trademark a plant, therefore the need to isolate the most active ingredient within the plant material is used today. When looking at the medicine-making industry as a whole, the basis is isolating compounds of highly medicinal plants, only to trademark the product and attach a very high dollar amount. This process leaves behind the automatic buffers mother nature has given to humanity, so we do not have negative side effects.

Long term use or high dosage of protein has been linked to the following, as per Livestrong the International School of Healing Arts and the International College of Holistic Studies:

Weight gain

Insulin exhaustion

Digestion problems

Kidney stones

Trace amount of heavy metals

Gout

Kidney disease

Organ failure

Kidney stones

Osteoporosis

Cancer

Toxicity

Protein supplements create a nitrogen by-product that kidneys have to work to filter out of the blood. With normal amounts of protein, we urinate out the nitrogen. But, with excessive protein, the kidneys have to work really hard to release the extra nitrogen, and over time, kidney hardship or damage can result. In facial body reading, the kidney connection is linked to the area under the eyes, and when this is dark or puffy, the remedy is in the kidney(s).

Also, dehydration can occur, because the body uses more water to flush excess protein.

Too much protein can make you gain weight when used long-term. In the short term, high protein may release unwanted weight, but when cutting out other foods (such as whole carbs and grains), you can gain weight. In a long-term study of 7000 adults, 90% who ate mostly protein became overweight due to the unbalance of fiber and protein, causing nutrient deficiency while missing the plant carbohydrate and fiber balance.

Also, isolated compounds are devoid of nutritional alkalizing minerals, which are naturally occurring vitamins, are lost in processing. This renders the supplement deficient and over-acidifying, which leads to muscle and bone tissue loss as the blood acidity rises.

It has also been noted that with excess protein, the G.I. tract becomes slow and has sluggish elimination. When our focus is on protein, we tend to forget other valuable nutrients like fiber (25 to 35 grams a day) and complex carbs (whole grains and beans, soaked or sprouted is best). With sluggish elimination, we can make way for yeast overgrowth, diverticulitis, feeling bloated, and inflammation. The link with the G.I. tract and sluggish elimination is low fiber intake. We can also be at risk for hyper amino academia (excess amino acids), hyper ammonia (excess ammonia), or hyper insulinemia nausea (excess insulin), giving way to organ failure and possible early death.

The body will convert most of the un-utilized calories of excess protein into sugar rather than fat. This allows for increased blood sugar levels that can feed bacteria and yeast candida, as well as fueling cancer cell growth, as sugar feeds cancer.

The recommended protein intake for women is 46 grams per day (while pregnant it's 25% more), and for men it is 56 grams per day, and rarely over 70 grams, which would be for a man working out 7 to 8 hours a day, such as a body builder. Most Americans eat over 100 grams of protein a day with just the Standard American Diet (SAD).

Best Whole Food Proteins - Living Vibrational Foods:

Soaked or sprouted will increase the nutrients and are easier to digest.

HEMP SEEDS	-	33% protein, 20 amino acids, and very easily digestible - loaded with omega 3 fats
CHIA SEEDS	-	14% protein - high in omega 3
SPIRULINA	-	70% protein - 4x more than red meat - 18 amino acids, easily assimilated iodine source (seafood allergy) - frequently used by vegan body builders
SPROUTS	-	Quality protein and fiber - beans, nuts, seeds, and grains
SUNFLOWER SPROUT	-	Highest quality protein found with iron and chlorophyll
KAMUT - HEMP - QUINOA	-	are all great sources

BEE POLLEN   -   known as a complete food - 40% protein and a full spectrum of nutrients - use in smoothies or on top of grain cereal

* * * *

When we choose foods that are good for us, we must keep everything in balance and not over consume them. For instance, just because oranges are good for you doesn't mean you should eat 10 of them in one day if you feel you may be catching a cold. That would create too much Vitamin C and acidity, which can give women a u.t.i., and would definitely give me a u.t.i. Variety is the spice of life and gives the body an opportunity to receive different nutrients within a "Whole food diet". Let's spice it up.

Books for reference on diet: *Macrobiotic Diet,* Micho Kushi; *Food for Life,* Seymour Koblin. *My Beautiful Life,* Mina Dobic. *Hip Chicks Guide to Macrobiotics,* Jessica Porter. With raw juicing there are so many recipes out there, just think green and enjoy.

"Anger is Contagious - Hate is Contagious - Jealousy is Contagious - Comparison is Contagious - Love is Contagious - What do You Want to Catch?"

-Miguel Ruiz

"I agree to win over fear and have the courage to face the truth."

-Miguel Ruiz

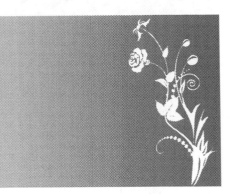

CHAPTER 4

Relax & Assimilate

"When we accept our own behavior to become the creator of our own disease, we can then change such behavior to achieve a desired outcome."

Rhea Iris Rivers

The next step was holding myself accountable and shifting from the inner-judge (ego), the critic holding me hostage. When we admit our short comings which create our health crisis, only then can we feel the empowerment of choice. The empowerment of choice fuels the energy needed for change. With this new-found energy, I realized that if *I can create a malignant growth within my own body, then the options for creation are limited to my own self-beliefs of what I feel I am worthy.* When I released the inner-judge by not acting on those thoughts and began to work within the present moment, I felt my vibration shift. I stepped into the most powerful version of myself yet.

I continued my research into the power of our thoughts and how they absolutely affect our health. Louise Hay created an empire on the topic and I have read many of her books and those of Hay House authors Don Miguel Ruiz, Doreen Virtue, Wayne Dyer, Denise Linn, Colette Baron-Reid, Bruce Lipton, and David Ji. I began taking workshops and absorbing Hay House books near the end of my marriage. I found these authors to be a powerful tool in reflection work and self-healing. But my diagnosis was a call to look at myself with new eyes and at deeper depths than I had in the past. A new perspective was at hand. I continued with my research.

Passion for nutritional healing ignites:

During my first nutrition class at the School of Healing Arts, Macrobiotics with Mina Dobic, author of *My Beautiful Life*, I heard the most unbelievable stories of healing. This class forever changed the way I look at foods, energy, stress, and self-healing. Her personal story of healing from metastasized cancer (more than one time), after being given a few months to live, is unbelievable. If you are fortunate enough to hear her story with your own ears and feel her passion for helping those in need, it truly was a pivotal point in my life. In Mina's journey, she walked out of her doctor's office and refused chemo or radiation (again), feeling that there must be a better way - listening to her inner guidance. It was then that her path to healing appeared: macrobiotics. This amazing woman changed the way she looked at cancer, began a completely new way of eating, found her purpose in life, and connected to the vibration of nature.

One of the students sitting next to me during her class was a young girl with M.S. Mina was her wellness consultant. She stated that before she found Mina she was taking enough medications to fill a bucket. She felt helpless and hopeless at nineteen years of age. She was then 24 and had shifted her M.S. into full remission with macrobiotics and Mina, and no longer needed the medications. I remember thinking: "This is crazy, a bunch of B.S." (Remember me, unawake in the early 2000s,) I said out loud "If changing our diet can heal cancer and M.S., then why doesn't anyone know about this way of healing?" in a snide tone. I felt the entire class turn to look at me as though I had grown a horn and must have been a Unicorn for a brief moment in time. In response, the students said "It is because there isn't any money in it." This way of thinking was considered way out there back in those days. In 2018 we can find pockets of the population that have shifted consciousness and are open to change, knowing we must start within ourselves. We can also find pockets of the population where change is still the enemy and who will resist change until lights out or the last tree stands.

During this course I also met two women who had breast cancer and chose to "change" their lifestyle, career, outlook on life, and viewed their own kitchens as medicine cabinets. Both women retained their breasts and fought off cancer, giving the new lifestyle of macrobiotics much gratitude.

As I neared the completion of these programs my level of confidence or lack thereof (in becoming an alternative wellness consultant) was extremely low. After being witness to such amazing transformations, how would I ever be able to be successful? After all, my attraction to alternative healing was ADHD and although difficult, is treatable and rather easy in comparison to cancer and auto-immune disorders. Fear and self-doubt sat within as I tried to imagine myself a wellness guru, which are the same emotions cancer is rooted in. Deep down within myself, for a brief moment, this thought entered my mind: "It would help if I had my own story of healing." Well, watch what you wish for, as those thoughts are mega powerful. It appears I again have a self-fulfilled prophecy.

I believe with all my heart that we become our thoughts: physically, emotionally, and spiritually. My lack of confidence carried into the later part of my nutritional counselor and herbalist programs as I dripped with fear and self-doubt.

During my case studies, I had amazing results with thyroid (hypo and hyper) disorders, candida, and clearing cancerous debris of the lymph system. With disruptions of the thyroid there is a connection to metal toxicity, which will give host to candida and other parasites (discussed within the Apothecary, under Folklore), a full clean-out was recommended. After the completion of the clean out, only then are tonic (long-term) herbs recommended. *When dealing with disruptions of the auto-immune system there is a connection to the emotional body, meaning, the immune system essentially turns on itself. The immune system becomes confused and attacks both healthy cells and foreign rogue intruder cells. This error in communication is linked to how the individual truly feels about themselves. If your inner-self is continually depleting your vibrational frequency by believing you are too fat, too poor, your nose is too big, you are awful in social settings, too short, too tall, not good enough, etc., I believe you get the picture. At this level of negativity the immune system identifies all cells being equals as they vibrate at the same rate. In a state of confusion, the immune system then begins to consume the healthy cells. This diagnosis is a cordial invitation to look at yourself with new eyes, and with a deeper perspective. Use variables A through Z if necessary to find what is no longer serving your best self.*

Regardless of my success with my case studies, I continued to feel less than confident as I entered the last part of these programs. I was having difficulty releasing past opinions and judgments on the healing arts. Coming out of a community in which the only way to heal was the MD or western medicine, where a naturopath doctor was also belittled and ridiculed, I lacked the confidence to stand for what I believed in. *But things were about to change.*

I would like to share a few stories of healing:

The following client received three reiki sessions with energy balancing and the release of congested energy. By releasing congested energy, you open pathways and increase the vibrational frequency of your entire system, giving way to healing not only vaginal cancer but all disease. Nutritional guidance and herbal recommendations were also given, taking approximately two and half months.

Alternative Wellness Client I:

I worked with Jane Doe in 2015, and she had *chronic candida and HPV with abnormal cell growth.* We cleared her of all complaints and received a clean test from her doctor. Jane had been seen by other nutritionists and her own MD and ND, and they could not clear her infestation of candida or the virus. I believe it is because none of the above-mentioned were herbalists. When dealing with a parasite like candida, western medications can not touch or destroy this intruder, as these parasites have a tolerance to antibiotics. Change of diet will slow them down but not evict them from the body. In fact, this parasite laughs, as it is a bully, and not to be taken lightly. I write more about this in the Apothecary section, under Folklore. Using our herbal allies, a virus can be minimized and cast from the body. Using the right plant and the right dosage is pure magic. Using the correct herbal ally at the correct dosage is imperative for beneficial results. *Always seek the advice of a certified herbalist when using our plant kingdom medicinally.*

Jane also had vaginal suppositories recommended (formula in the Apothecary section; under fine china suppository), medicinal herbal teas and supplements, bowel cleanser, probiotics, and flower essence.

In May of 2017 Jane received another normal result from a colposcopy test. Go Jane.

Alternative Wellness Client II

Jane Doe II arrived in June of 2016. She had a diagnosis of *VAIN 3, severe dysplasia with active HPV.* The protocol was three energy sessions, nutritional guidance, vaginal suppositories, medicinal herbal teas and supplements, bowel cleanser, probiotics, and flower essence. She received a clean exam report in August of 2016, also a clean exam in July of 2017 and is almost due for her 2018 annual. Way to go Jane II, keep up the good work.

Alternative Wellness Client III:

John Doe came to me with a horrible *staph infection* inside his nose. He had been on two rounds of antibiotics and received no relief from the infection, as the bacteria had built up a tolerance to antibiotics. He was entering heavy stress, high panic mode while this bacteria stood its ground. This particular staph infection was known for being intelligent, and was able to re-establish its dominance very quickly. When working topically with this type of bacteria it is important to not only treat the flesh but the inner workings of the anatomy.

Recommended as oral supplements were astragalus root (highlighted within the Apothecary, under oral supplements and vaginal suppository) and kick-ass biotic by Wishgarden Herbs (highlighted within the Apothecary, under dog meat: Usnea lichen, bee propolis, myrrh gum, goldenseal root, baptisia root, red root, hops strobiles, boneset aerials, echinacea angustifolia root, echinacea purpurea root) and raw garlic.

Topically, we mixed ancient healing clay, garlic, burdock root, colloidal silver, manuka honey, oil of oregano and turmeric. We removed all sugar from his diet, even kombucha. Other dietary changes and distant healings were given. The recommended dosage was every 1 to 3 hours for 14 days, astragalus was taken long term, and the topical formula was applied many times a day for the maximum time allowed.

The *staph infection* was no match for mother nature, and admitted defeat. *Staph* is very stubborn and not to be taken lightly. When bacteria finds a way to survive by building a tolerance to an antibiotic, please ask Gaia for assistance.

When working with our plant kingdom herbal allies, it is important to understand the more the merrier (within reason) as plants work synergistically and communicate on a level we are just beginning to understand. Working with blended tinctures is a wonderful way to ensure the correct amount of each herbal ally is part of the formulation. Please leave the blending to the Master

Herbalists, as some plants are born to work with certain plants and need the ancient knowledge of the masters.

While I maintain the research detective within, the journey into myself was just getting juicy. With a lightened heart and unsure of a positive outcome, I continued my quest for more knowledge and kept the positive vibe flowing. The colposcopy appointment was on the horizon, and I had much work to do.

Catalyst for change:

I have noticed when working with wellness clients, the clients that have the most difficultly promoting change in their daily routines are the exact clients who are unable to quiet the mind chatter and hear inner-guidance. They just "can't" meditate. There is frequently a correlation between the person with spinning mind and digestive issues. When digestive issues become a common trait in a person, the rest of the body begins to suffer. The body shows signs of immune system dysfunction, respiratory system dysfunction, cardio vascular system dysfunction, nervous system dysfunction, musculoskeletal system dysfunction, endocrine system dysfunction, and reproductive system issues. The spinning mind and endless chatter is the foundation for our stress response or the fight or flight response.

Becoming the observer of the endless stream of thoughts, rather than the performer of every thought, is the result of a trained mind. Although these clients truly do want change, they continue their lives of jumping from one performance to the next, being controlled by endless stream of thoughts or circular thinking. During meditation, the practice is placing each entering thought to the side and refocusing on the desired goal of the meditation, repeatedly. It sounds simple because it is, and it is absolutely free, effective, and vibrationally up-lifting. ***Meditation trains the brain the way exercise trains the body, by repetition.*** By doing this five to ten minutes each day, you will notice a shift. The body will recede from the fight or flight response with simple daily meditations.

With meditation, some may be able to handle anger with a softer approach. Some may be able to release thoughts of depression as these thoughts keep one locked in the past. Some may be able to slow a racing, anxiety-filled heart by continuously re-centering in the present tense. And some may notice when their thoughts have jumped into future tense, assuming a future outcome when there is no way of knowing that outcome and creating distress rather than body-reading and finding their solution.

Thoughts enter throughout the day, and one can choose to observe the passing thought or become the performer of every thought, *like a teenager.* This is a choice and choices are made in the present tense and in complete empowerment.

Happiness is a choice, Happenings always happen, your choice which direction to go. -Miguel Ruiz

Breathe and release, relax and assimilate:

Learning to meditate has been hands down the most rewarding and least expensive symptom relief I have ever experienced. When you come to a place in your meditation exercise of true silence, where the break in chatter exists, that is where your inner-guidance is heard. How are you able to know whether you heard inner-guidance? Inner-guidance could be something you've never realized before that moment, or a thought you have known all along but had stuffed too deeply within yourself. Inner-guidance should give you feelings of elation, connectedness, and inspire you to understand yourself on a deeper, more compassionate level. Inner-guidance should give you a feeling of connectedness to all living things, bringing joy to those around you.

I attended a course offered by Hay House, called The Art of Meditation, by David Ji. I found it to be very simple to follow, and would like to share some of the highlights.

The *fight or flight response* is a bit of a buzz word now, but this does not make it any less real or dangerous. If you remember the truth about coffee from the last chapter, read the following knowing that this is what you go through with each cup of java. Here is what happens when the body shifts into stress mode or fight or flight.

Your body instinctively begins to perspire, and depending on your chosen diet, this "sweat" can be really stinky. Odor will fluctuate upon your level of toxicity.

You may begin to breathe more quickly, which will increase your blood flow, blood pressure, pulse, and stress on your heart.

The pulsing blood moves into your muscles so you can either run away or battle for your life. The body does not know the difference between a scary movie or a missed deadline at work. This response is automatic.

As the blood flow moves into your extremities, the blood leaves your organs and your digestive tract, leaving any undigested food in the gut, slowing your metabolism and weakening the surrounding tissue. It's no wonder why so many Americans have leaky gut syndrome.

The stress hormones cortisol, adrenaline, and glucagon start to surge, giving extra energy and focus to escape the unknown danger.

Your pancreas slows insulin production and your blood sugar spikes.

Your body shuts down all functions not essential for the fight or flight response, i.e., growth hormone (hair, nails, skin, cellular development) and sex hormones including the reproductive system. Here we find the link to coffee consumption and fertility.

Your immune system shuts down, as it is not necessary when you are running for your life or fighting for your life. You may die at any moment.

Your blood becomes thick and sticky. Your body believes it maybe cut and starts to clot in advance.

Over time, this repeated exposure leaves you vulnerable to illness, i.e., IBS, Crohn's disease, migraine headaches, skin disorders, PTSD, premature aging, skin dryness, hormone disruptions, early menopause, and cancer. The emotional vulnerability is also real, such as shutting down vocally, becoming overreactive, aggressive, or physically abusive. These are a few issues that can develop, but the F or F response is the butterfly which affects our entire existence.

Once the stress hormones have been released, there is no off switch for cortisol. Cortisol surges within the body for hours after its release. When there are prolonged levels of cortisol within the blood stream, the body begins to suffer:

Decreased bone density
Lock of focus
Thyroid function imbalance
Increased blood pressure
Blood sugar imbalance
Increased abdominal fat
Suppressed immune system
Suppressed inflammatory response
Hippocampus shrinks, affecting memory, new brain cell development, and the ability to learn
Increased amygdala size, keeping us in fear-based learning mode, where we are unable to hear our inner-guidance

Meditation and the fight or flight response:
How does meditation become part of the fight or flight response? Meditation has been proven to counter the stress response. Isn't that amazing? When our body is able to be the observer rather than the performer of every thought that comes to mind, the entire system shifts to a place of higher vibration, giving way to less mental and physical illness. Daily meditation brings calmness, making us less reactive, less angry, more patient, more creative, and full of gratitude, joy, and generosity. We begin to flow in our life rather than our life banging us around on its own journey.

During meditation the following occurs:

Breath is quiet and more relaxed
Heart rated decreases, easing our blood pressure
Digestive systems returns to normal and blood returns
Cortisol, adrenalin, glucagon - stress hormones slow their surges
Immune system begin to function
Blood becomes less sticky and flows freely
Mode of learning returns to the expansiveness of a child
Ability to focus improves, ability to learn improves, memory improves

To begin, simply check in with yourself. What are you feeling? Breathe a few deeps breaths in with a full exhale. The intention is to interrupt the fight or flight response, and is very simple yet effective. You are demanding control of your mind, body, and spirit.

On the breath, breathe in, hold full, breathe out, hold empty. Do this a few times, until you feel the release. Pay attention to how the air feels flowing from the nose into the lungs and back up the throat to the nose. This can be done while sitting on the toilet, or in your car while picking up your kids. Breath work is the foundation, and can realign a spinning, anxiety-filled mind to a relaxed introspective state. It is free, has zero interactions with medications, and feels great.

Once you've mastered the breath work and tuning in, you can easily move into deeper meditations. Choose a word for a focus point (for example, gratitude) and when anything other than gratitude enters your mind, place the thought to the side, and continue with what you are grateful for. Repeat. Easy peasy and effective.

As a current reiki usui master/karuna holy fire II master/teacher, the very first level of reiki we learn: to know thyself is to heal thyself. We are also taught at this level that the practitioner is not the healer, but rather a loving guide and a channel for healing energy. The client and the energy itself are the healers.

With my colposcopy on the horizon, I felt the need for spiritual guidance. I turned to the healing method that is always available for me, rain or shine, here or there: meditation and reiki, which are my favorite. One could be naked on the highest point of planet earth and have the ability to channel reiki energy, or, god forbid, in jail. Energy healing can be used by anyone, no matter the diagnosis or which planet they are from. It is safe and enormously effective.

Meditation and reiki were a big part of my road to recovery. I performed self treatments on a daily basis, more than once a day, and often more than three times a day. I believe the more energy workers there are on the planet, the more amazing the planet will be. I would love to see alternative education become part of the high school curriculum. Imagine if lifting vibrations and expanding knowledge of oneself was widespread, this would nourish our entire country. During meditations, I received guidance to trust in what I had studied. Although I do not have a PhD behind my name, the "hippie dippie" education I love so much has great value, not just for my benefit, but for the benefit of those who seek the same knowledge. The true benefit lies with honoring our Gaia, our forgotten allies, and that which gives life. Caring for the soil and all the beautiful organisms which live beneath it is of major concern, and another reason to become a conscious consumer. Conscious consuming is caring to purchase items for the betterment of society, for further generations and mother nature, versus one's own self gratification.

During this special time of meditation, I would escape outdoors, find Gaia in her glory, take off my shoes to feel the earth, and breathe. I felt a sense of interconnectedness to all energetic beings and knew that I was never alone. Also, I felt now is the time to use my voice and speak of experiences different than most without fear of ridicule. To trust in the process of life, knowing this is part of my journey and necessary to release residual thoughts of fear. To shift to a space of surrender and trust. In the tranquil space of surrender, inner-guidance is plentiful. When we are able to feel the heart expand in gratitude for life's road bumps and come to a space of complete relaxation, we can then begin the process of healing in its entirety.

Benefits of Reiki:

Reiki allows for the clearing of blocked vibrational frequency, therefore, increasing our vibrational frequency +MHz. Reiki energy is channeled through the practitioner into the client. The practitioner holds their hands over different parts of the body for three minutes to much longer, depending on what the client needs.

Many of these points during application of Reiki are linked with our endocrine system. This system is responsible for many job duties, one of which is the ability to balance the continued release of the fight or flight response. As the exhaustion of the endocrine system settles into our daily lifestyle, we can become host to many crises, including hormonal disturbances, sleep disturbances and emotional turmoil. These disturbances also include thyroid disorders to reproductive system failure. Reiki allows the body *in it's entirety* to release stress and begin to rebuild from exhaustion. **A state of complete relaxation is the only space where the body is able to heal.**

Reiki allows one to gain greater clarity when dealing with life lessons. When dealing with depression Reiki allows the vibrational frequency to rise, giving way to the release of our happy hormones.

Reiki has also been known to assist with better focus and the ability to stay in the present moment. Reiki can bring on the ease of falling asleep and staying asleep. Reiki helps heal inflammation and infection. Reiki can reduce the effects of heart disease and other chronic conditions. Reiki has been used to reduce pain from arthritis or migraines, and assist with cancer in treating fatigue, pain, and depression.

"Just for today, I will let go of anger, I will let go of worry. Today, I will count my many blessings. Today, I will do my work honestly. Today, I will be kind to every living creature."

-Mikao Usui
(said daily, with gassho hand position
meditation, in reiki practice)

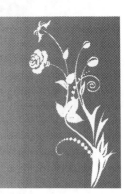

CHAPTER 5

Beautiful Communication

"I agree to use my words in order to create a better world, not just for myself, but for the generations to come."

-Miguel Ruiz

As I searched for more knowledge the connection to communication and the growth of cancer cells had a connection. Throughout my life I have communicated on a level which is conducive to the level of my success within my relationships. My communication has been passive-aggressive, or just plain aggressive. When communicating in passive-aggressive mode, I believed the recipient should have the ability to read my mind or read between the lines, or understand what I was truly trying to communicate without ever using the proper words. Then, out of frustration of not being understood, I would slip into aggressive communication. I was a ticking time bomb. I believe this part of my research was to bring me to an authentic level, allowing me to use words that matched my true emotions, giving way to success on every level and benefitting those around me. Beautiful communication equals beautiful life and nourishes the relationship of self-love.

I was fortunate to find a course by Doreen Virtue called Assertiveness Communication. I would like to share some of the highlights that transformed my way of thinking about communication. This course was literally an answer to my prayers. I was having difficulty relaying verbal messages to clients after reiki treatments and during consultations. Part of my block at that time was learning to trust my inner-voice, and the other part was knowing proper word usage and tone while relaying messages.

Beautiful assertive communication:

Have you ever felt invisible while speaking to a group? Or have you felt so strongly about your opinion that you disregarded the feelings of others? I have, and if you have, then you are among the majority of the population. You may have felt that a different approach would better serve you. But which approach? Most communication styles fluctuate between passive-aggressive and aggressive expression. With the popularity of reality television and our news media, which capitalizes on these forms of communication, the ability to speak lovingly and assertively is a life skill we must seek to learn. I most definitely had to seek to learn the rudiments.

To communicate assertively is to express your feelings in a loving, honest, and direct manner. Sound easy? Expressing yourself assertively allows others to have different opinions, without feeling upset, offended, or believing that your view is the only right position. Again, just watch our news media or reality TV and notice how the communication of the public begins to mirror these outlets.

To be truly assertive, you know who you are, acknowledge your heartfelt truth (even if you are not proud of it), and are on target to living your deepest dreams. Assertive communication is not about changing other people, it is about positive self-expression and the ability to listen. While you listen you have the ability to repeat words you have heard to ensure clear communication. This is very difficult for some people, including me sometimes. Looking at the current state of America, where most are concerned with their opinion being heard, and believe that opinion is the only correct one, the inability to listen is disastrous and reduces vibrational frequency as a nation. In my opinion, we as a nation need to work on our assertiveness communication to begin to lift one another up.

To communicate in an aggressive manner is to verbalize your feelings so strongly that you disregard the feelings of others. Aggressive communication disregards other views as having zero value, as you believe your way is the only way. Basically, the bully is born. When aggressive communication is being used, many people may be offended and even emotionally or physically wounded by your words and or actions. This form of communication can be rooted in fear due to feelings of your own inadequacies. I have expressed myself aggressively. Have you?

To communicate with a passive-aggressive tone is to use words in a roundabout form to express yourself. You may be unable to truly connect and express your feelings and emotions, keeping them hidden, and use communication tools like sarcasm or humor to engage in meaningful conversation. This form of communication may also be rooted in fear due to low self-worth or a shattered belief in self. I have expressed myself passive-aggressively. Have you?

After reviewing the different ways of communication, which type do you see yourself using? Once you have the visual, bring your attention to your childhood, and examine which type of communication your family used in conversation. We are usually a mix between the two parent figures. How do you wish to be viewed as a communicator? When I looked back in my life, I most definitely flowed between the two extremes, a blend of the middle-child with aggressive communication and passive-aggressive communication sharing the spotlight. It is important to *not* feel guilt about past communication behaviors, but rather except the lesson in gratitude and grow for the experience. Would you feel while communicating in a non-assertive manner, your vibrational frequency would rise or begin to fall? Bingo, it would fall.

Another important part of this course was being able to view myself with new eyes. A new perspective entered my life in a huge way. Learning the rudiments of boundaries, co-dependency, people-pleasing, rescue addiction, and being the victim. As I said before, this course was an answer to my prayers. I believe the gift of a new perspective is the basis of all change, and without change, things remain the same. If I have a disgusting malignant growth, why would I want things to remain unchanged?

Boundaries - Tool for self-care. We have a right to our own thoughts, time, and space. As an entrepreneur, I frequently changed my personal schedule to please a client. I no longer do so. When the phone rings many times it goes to voicemail and the call is returned on my schedule. I trust all time will be available when desired and released the need to control. Do you feel my personal power soaring?

Co-Dependency - I will only be happy if you are happy. I will do anything to make you happy, then detach emotionally. Staying in unhealthy relationship past expiration. Yes, I can see past patterns to this one, but this is also behind me.

People Pleasing - One who gives of themselves fully, lacks substance, has no opinion, never able to see the real person, and manipulates people with kindness for control over them. Yes, I can identify here too, occasionally.

Rescue Addiction – A pattern of relationships where you are clearly the rescuer, and the other person is the victim in need of rescuing. There could be food, chaos, financial or drug addictions. I attract this type of person and fortunately I am now able to identify very quickly, and move through it.

Victim - One who believes they do not participate in their misfortune, and does not take responsibly for life's mishaps. Yes, I can identify here, but this is also behind me.

Check in with yourself. Do any of these resonate in your life? To be assertive is to constantly check in with how people or situations make you feel. _To become in tune with how you feel is the best way to communicate on a direct level and feel the empowerment of voice_. I feel that boundary, co-dependency, people-pleasing, rescue addiction and being the victim resonated with me. It is only after recognizing personal patterns that we can re-write them.

Why would I choose to re-write what I believe is causing disharmony? I believe that if we do not work on these lessons in this life, the lesson is carried into future lives. Laugh if you will, and I realize it may be far-fetched, but why couldn't this be the way? If true, we will revisit the lesson until we process it, learn, and grow spiritually. Once we solidify the lesson, we raise our vibrational frequency, reduce physical and mental illness, and release the pattern of behavior. I think it is worth a try.

During this time in my life, I truly felt the saying: "When the Student is ready, the Master appears". One of my favorite roles in life has been being a student of life and a student in the classroom.

"If you lend your consciousness to someone else, you're a robot."

-Prince

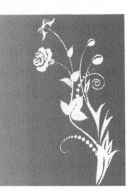

CHAPTER 6

Flowers Galore

"The quieter you become the more you are able to hear."

Rumi

The more I raised my vibrational frequency, the better I felt. Flower essence was a big part of helping me move through the rubbish I had created. Flower essences are in a league of their own. In ancient stories that pre-date our written history, flower essences were used in vibrational healing. This story begins in Lemuria, the ancient civilization from 4500,000 BC to 12,000 years ago. Lemuria is known as, "the lost land" and the "garden of Eden." During these ancient times, Lemurians were thought to live without disease in any form. Flower essences were used to promote spiritual consciousness. This allowed for the alignment between the emotional, physical, and spiritual bodies. The essence was known as "liquid consciousness," with the highest level of vibrational frequency found in the flower.

It is believed that when a body reaches its highest vibrational frequency, this plateau is where optimum health exists. Free from emotional distress, the body and spirit are left in a state of freeness and tranquility, without disease. Can you imagine? It sounds like "the garden of Eden." This knowledge is believed to have been passed down to Atlantis, then into Egypt. There are hieroglyphics showing their adoration for the essence.

Let's visualize for a moment this entire planet during springtime, with flowers blooming at every turn, you can see how many flower varieties are available for mankind. Each flower has its own specific job duty. For instance:

St. Johns Wort (yellow) is known for releasing conscious and subconscious fear, bringing in belief of divine guidance and protection, and assisting in dealing with fearful dreams. While ingesting the essence, you repeat its affirmation or one which feels best to you. St. Johns Wort affirmation: I trust the divine spirit to know my inner light as a source of guidance and protection. I am courageous in both waking and dream life.

Pomegranate essence is known to free the feminine creative energy (in men and women), finding how to express one's creativity, helping to transform emotions relating to lack of childhood nurturance. Affirmation: I nurture seed ideas, and give birth to creative expression. I am nurtured by the universal love of the divine mother principle.

The many flower essence qualities and affirmations can be found online. During my flower essence course, The Flowers Essence Society (FES), were spoken of highly within most of the material presented. Dr. Bach Flower Essences were also part of the course, and can generally be found at Sprouts.

What is a Flower Essence? How do Flower Essence, Essential Oils, and Tinctures differ?

Flower essence treats the emotional body, which affects our physical body. Tinctures and essential oils treat the physical body, which affect our emotional body. There is some overlap of treatment, but that is a good starting point. Flower essences were believed to be rediscovered by Dr. Bach in the 1930s. The use of the essence had been forgotten until Dr. Bach discovered that the dew on flower petals held healing properties, and found a way to recreate what Gaia had already designed. Each flower has a specific duty, just as each herbal ally or each person has a duty. This magical elixir helps us balance negative attitudes and feelings, see life in different perspectives, and allows our life to shift. Flower essences are odorless, unlike essential oils, and specialize in harmonizing the emotional body.

The essence or energetic character is captured in water, glycerin, or an alcohol solution with very little plant material, unlike an essential oil. When this magical elixir is made, human hands never touch the flowers, instead, the leaves of other plants, i.e., mullein leaves, cover hands during production. This practice is to ensure the vibrational level of the person does not transfer to the liquid, keeping it pure. These vibrant champions of Gaia raise our vibrational frequency. I used a few different flower essences before and during my healing phase, as well as currently. I took four drops per day, four times per day (sometimes more or less) and repeated an affirmation. You can also rub it onto your lips, or place drops behind your ears, temples, and wrist.

My first choice was wild oat. I began taking this solution months before my diagnosis, as I felt the need for an energetic shift. I did not take it regularly, just when I remembered. Wild oat is for a person who is unsure of making decisions, or ready for change and not sure which way to go. At the time, I didn't feel a shift, but now as I write these words I feel wild oat was working at a level so deep that it was difficult to see in the moment. I am no longer working on the inability to make decisions. I'm working on something else: "After climbing a great hill… one only finds there are many more hills to climb."

Around the time of my diagnosis, I tried a second essence, gentian, and I instantly felt a shift: the feeling of butterflies in my stomach, and pure excitement. Gentian is for a person who becomes easily discouraged when things go wrong, and has lack of strength to accomplish goals. If you are reading this book, it means that I completed this book, so gentian showed up and did its job. "She believed she could, so she did."

Making a flower essence at home can be as easy as putting rose petals in your water and allowing the glass jar to sit in the sun or full moon for a few hours, then drink. Of course, the rose must never have been sprayed with pesticides and was hopefully grown without chemical fertilizers. Easy peasy. For a full guide on how to make flower essence, refer to James Green's book.

Currently, or at the time of writing this book, I am taking flower essence of mullein. Magical mullein is known for having a combination of courage and tenderness while facing one's own fears. It aligns our physical body with our emotional body, and is very grounding. It allows for a solid moral conscience and strong feelings of truthfulness. Would you say mullein has had a profound effect of my writing? I believe so.

During the writing phase I also took the tincture "Genius Juice," from Wishgarden Herbs. This tincture is brain food and helps with everything from jet lag, studying, ADHD, failing memory, and hangovers. The herbal allies are gotu kola, ginko, eleuthero root, dandelion root, cinnamon bark, and prickly ash bark. Truly a remarkable formula, it helps the brain kick it in high gear, without the use of caffeine or expelling the adrenals. Genius juice is great for the person attempting to kick the coffee addiction, safely and without the release of the flight or fight response.

There are dozens of flower essences just waiting for you. They are safe, with no known interactions, and are very affordable. What's stopping you? Maybe fear has edged its way into your mind? Let's check in with ourselves. Close your eyes and breathe a full breath, hold at the top, release, and hold at the bottom, release. Search your emotions. Does this fear have anything to do with someone being witness to you consuming such a hippie dippie health alternative? Have you ever laughed at or disregarded alternative healing? Do you live in a community where alternative healing is cast as a joke? If you said yes to any of these, then it is possible fear is delaying your transition.

Daily affirmations:

Louise Hay said it so beautifully with a daily affirmation: "I am not responsible for other people. We are all under the law of our own consciousness." Basically, the message is - you do you and I'll do me - or - mind your own affairs. If a certain path is calling one to journey, one should be able to travel without fear of belittlement. If one feels this may be the current situation, then looking for a broader community may be in the future. When we move fear from our passenger seat to the back seat, we open ourselves to a new on-board passenger of our choosing. I chose my new passenger to be support, which was found in a "broader community." Who will you choose?

Along with flower essence, I chose positive affirmations like "I love my body," "my voice matters," "I love unconditionally," "my body is vibrantly healthy," and said them aloud 10,000'ish times a day. These affirmations were written on post-it notes and placed on my car dash, my work space, and the bathroom mirror to ensure my train of thought remained on the positive side of the tracks.

Louise Hay has a annual calendar, and each day she has written a beautiful affirmation which I use frequently as a focus point for daily meditations. I love this one: "I create easily and effortlessly when I let my thoughts come from the loving space of my own heart," or this one: "The more grateful I am, the more good experiences float my way," or this one: "I have more than enough time to do everything I want. Time expands for me." They are incredible, are they not? Do you feel lighter, an expansion of breath, after reading affirmations? I do.

Energetic body:

The energetic blueprint of a human body has several different layers. Beginning at the most dense of all the bodies is the physical body. You are able to see, touch, and smell in this body. The physical body is also known as the etheric body, and energetically, it goes beyond the skin one to three inches, and can have varying tones of color depending upon your level of health and vibrational frequency. These colors are able to be photographed with Kirlian photography, for the more science-minded individuals or those who would just enjoy a cool picture of their vibrational frequency. The emotional body expands one to two inches further than the physical body. This energetic body is known as your aura. All bodies can receive, give, and emit their own vibrational frequency. For the purpose of this book, I have mostly focused on the physical and emotional bodies. Beyond the emotional body are the spiritual planes which are interesting to research if you feel called to do so.

"The first law of thermodynamics doesn't actually specify that matter can be neither created nor destroyed, but instead that the total amount of energy in a closed system cannot be created nor destroyed (though it can be changed from one form to another)."

We are all matter. All matter contains energy. Energy cannot be seen. Energy is not only in matter, it is interdependent in creating universal order. When universal order is obtained, the vibrational frequency is higher. With universal order, we can then evolve into conscious consuming and thinking of others as well as ourself, thus evolving into compassion for all life including mother nature. Then we can evolve into the highest levels of joy, community, and generosity.

"When we look at our being as a vibrational space, all levels of healing are then obtainable."

- Rhea Iris Rivers

CHAPTER 7

I'm Coming Out

"Look for the Woman in the Dress. If there is no
Woman, there is no dress."

-Coco Chanel

Physical movement played a role in my healing phase. I chose not to
over-burden my body with heavy physical demands, which would
trigger flight or fight response, but rather to find nourishing ways
to balance my systems. Also, I chose chiropractic and massage
treatments to further the movement of my vibrational frequency.

Yoga was part of my program. I chose mostly outdoor yoga, and
used a towel as my mat. By using a towel I was able to receive and
transfer energy from the sun into the earth. Rubber mats act as an
energetic block to the flow of energy. Yoga has been part of my life
for many years, but during the time leading up to my diagnosis,
I was not exercising very much. After my diagnosis, I began my
exercise regimen again, attending yoga classes a few times a week,
and throwing a spin class into the mix occasionally. Spin class is a
great way to remove toxins from the lungs and the breath. It moves

the circulatory system and allows for the cleaning of the blood and lymph fluid. Both yoga and spin are known to move stuck energy and blockages, allowing for higher vibration.

Yoga is an ancient art with many benefits. It helps with flexibility and reduces pain in muscles and joints, helping with arthritis and back pain. It builds strong muscles and assists with perfect body posture. It reduces the chance of injury in daily life, prevents cartilage and joint breakdown while keeping the spine flexible, and straightens and strengthens vertebrae. Yoga increases blood flow and aids organs in detoxification. It regulates adrenal glands and allows the body to rest and digest, reducing the fight or flight response. It elevates mood and helps focus. It creates space in the lungs and can prevent IBS and digestive distress. Amazing, wouldn't you agree? Does this make you want to head out to a yoga or spin class?

While taking time daily for meditations and attending yoga class outside, I was able to increase my vitamin D, which is a very important part of healing. Low vitamin D is linked to cancer. When we raise vitamin D, it has been found to decrease our risk of cancer. Since many vitamin D supplements are synthetic, isolated, and lack vibrational frequency, I find it best to catch the early beauty of the champion of Mother Earth, the sun. Sunlight is known to increase serotonin levels and elevate your mood. Skin exposed to UV light will release nitric oxide, lowering blood pressure. Healthy levels of vitamin D have been linked with the prevention of: cancer, multiple sclerosis, and depression, and it promotes acceptable bone growth. The sun provides energy to generate life within our seas and on our land, giving energy to all plant and animal life on earth, and nourishing the many habitats on this beautiful rock.

I left no stone unturned while researching the cause of this disease. I changed my view of life, changed my diet, changed how I communicated, increased the frequency of my meditations and energy work, and found gratitude in every corner. It was now time for my colposcopy exam. I breathed deeply, many, many times as I arrived for the appointment.

Colposcopy Results:

It is time for the colposcopy. I enter the exam room, and find the same OB/GYN from my first exam, three weeks ago. This is the doctor who was called in for further assessment, the "colleague" who was needed for a second opinion. She is the one who stated: "I don't know what that is. Take a biopsy." She is very thorough in comforting me and explaining the colposcopy procedure. I assure her I am ready and say: "I'm a middle-aged woman with two children. This cannot be as painful as childbirth. Let's get on with it," with a snicker. With my feet in those oh-so-unwelcoming stirrups, the exam begins. What I hear next will live in my mind forever. She says, "You, You had lesions! You had growths! Your skin??? What did you do?! It's gone!" She exclaims as she stands from her stool to look down on my face. I say, "I felt as though it was gone. I couldn't feel anything any longer." Again, she exclaims, "What did you do?!" I explain that I am an "almost" herbalist and made herbal suppositories (found in the Apothecary) using turmeric, garlic, poke root…. reiki…. I notice her eyes glaze over and she sits back down on her stool to continue the exam, silently. I can only assume she cannot accept my hippie dippie education as having any real value or healing benefits, so she shut down, in a state of disbelief. Poor girl. But I feel the most unbelievable level of joy that I almost get up from the table and go home without completing the exam. But, of course I don't. I am just thinking cheap.

I eagerly awaited the test results, feeling certain I had cleared the accumulations, but then again, not entirely certain. These tests are an incredibly tool and the beauty of modern medicine.

Guess what? The test results came back clean and clear for malignant squamous cell accumulations and HPV. From the tone of the receptionist on the other end of the phone giving me my results, she was also in disbelief.

The time period was under 30-days. That's right. From pap diagnosis to colposcopy diagnosis. I was able to feed my entire being in a nourishing loving way, and in turn my body literally released all accumulations. I was so happy.

Do I believe these alternative healing modalities will cure all illness? No, I believe in the balance between allopathic and alternative healing modalities. Do I believe alternative healing modalities can be of benefit regardless of diagnosis? You betcha.

I also believe that sometimes people are called to cross over, and that passing with an illness where we know we are dying can be something to be grateful for. That may sound heartless, but none of us are getting out of here alive. I am not referring to a child, and send much love to those in that situation. If we know we are dying, we have the chance for closure with the people who mean the most to us. We also have the choice of making up with our arch enemy, if desired. We have the ability to forgive and hopefully to be forgiven. It is my belief that whatever we do not deal with in this life will carry over to our next life. The soul lesson is on repeat of the life lesson until we learn from the obstacle, and grow from its lesson.

How much are you grateful for?:

Gratitude is an emotion that was new to me before this life lesson and which I have struggled many times to reach. After this experience, my ability to reach gratitude has become a simpler task. I feel the more that I focus on things in my life that I'm grateful for, the more things I am grateful for. My daily struggles remain, as everyone has something they are dealing with. But after my struggles are handled, my focus returns to something I have learned from the struggle, which leads to more gratitude.

I purchased a wonderful tool that continues to lead me to new perspectives: a deck of cards called *Living Wisdom with his Holiness the Dalai Lama*. This incredible man is the vision of an egoless soul. He is without fear and has been able to maintain the beautiful curiosity of a child. I continually take a card from this deck to assist me in shifting my perception, and I would like to share a few messages that I found to be most inspiring:

"Giving is not merely a remedy against greed. The purpose of generosity is to increase the courage of giving. This is called the Transcendent Perfection of Generosity."

"If we forget ourselves in order to benefit others, if we are prepared to give our own lives to save the lives of others, and if we are giving them whatever is necessary for their welfare, then we shall gain happiness and all perfection."

"If you become proud and arrogant when giving, or if you practice generosity with the idea of a reward, then all the merit of the generosity is lost. Instead, pray that the positive karmic result of generosity will ripen in others rather than within ourselves."

Let's check in again with ourselves. How are you feeling? Does your heart feel full and spilling with emotions? My heart is feeling over-stuffed with the beauty of gratitude and generosity of mankind and I have a funny smile on my face. I focus daily on the beauty mankind has brought rather than the destruction, that way the flow of energy will increase the beauty of mankind. Where attention goes, energy flows.

The 7-Steps for Renewal

1. What's Your Frequency
   Where do you vibrate?
2. Emotional Awareness
   Which emotions resonate most?
3. Nutritional Guidance
   How well do you know your kitchen?
4. Relax and Assimilate
   Can you feel the breath moving?
5. Beautiful Communication
   How do you want your community to see you?

6. Flowers Galore
    Which essence fits you best?
7. I'm Stepping Out
    How much are you grateful for?

With these simple steps, I cleared a physical accumulation of a squamous cell malignancy and the HPV virus, in under 30-days. The depth of my cancerous growth is unknown because by the time the colposcopy appointment arrived, which would of identified the depth of the growth, I had cleared all accumulations of this disease. This left my doctor in total disbelief. I realize it can be scary to walk your own path and go against the grain as I have, but in reality, most of us will need to wait at least 30 days for an appointment to see whichever specialist is recommended after such a diagnosis. If we use the 30 days of waiting to self-evaluate and treat the body's vibrational frequency, it can only strengthen us. This allows for a stronger self if surgery or other treatment is still needed. But of course, the intention is to kick this issue out of the body by the time you reach your appointment. Positive vibes only.

In addition, after I received the clear colposcopy, I went for a routine visit with my chiropractor and acupuncturist (she is a double doctor and wonderful, Dr. Michele K. Ross, DC., of Tree of Life Chiropractic) which my body will yearn for at times. She asked me about the cyst I had on my middle right hand on the third knuckle. We had been watching the hideous lump at each appointment due to it's continuous growth. I had completely forgot the cyst until I was reminded, when I felt for the lump, there was no lump to be felt. It too had completely vanished. I smiled of course, and thought, never doubt the power of vibrational healing. I am never without amazement, the more I learn, the more I love.

"To become your own healer, you need only listen to your inner-voice."

-Rhea Iris Rivers

"Why do people say 'Grow some balls?' Balls are weak and sensitive! If you really wanna be tough, grow a vagina! Those things take a pounding!"

-Betty White

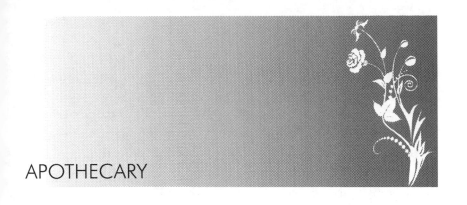

APOTHECARY

Introducing
Our Forgotten Allies

It is recommended to seek professional guidance when using our forgotten allies. The apothecary is NOT intended to diagnose a health crisis. The intention is to bring alternative views with the introduction of our forgotten allies.

Following are the herbal allies I used during the healing phase of my diagnosis and other ailments. But first, I feel compelled to share a memory. When I look back at memories during the time of my herbology courses, one story has remained vivid.

One of my instructors spoke of a time in the late 1800-1900s. A time when science and the very beginning of pharma were looking for a place to fit into the herbal wellness scene. The story went like this:

On the same night throughout the U.S., every herbal clinic was burned to the ground. The persons responsible were never brought to justice. Anyone having knowledge or practice of herbology was banished and accused of witchery and anyone who knew the said "witches" were also banished, or marked as outcasts.

Although these happenings were noted prior to the 1800-1900s, not only in the U.S. but in Europe, its been proven that the accused were at times burned alive. It was then that herbology was buried and practiced underground, out of fear of banishment or death. This abuse was in public areas for all to see. By holding public prosecution, it assured that deep-rooted fear was struck into the souls of everyone within the community. Fear is known to attach to DNA, and keeps one in fear-mode learning, reducing brain matter. The attachment to DNA is passed down through generations. Present day fear remains within our communities, keeping many from using our herbal allies for their own well-being. It has been proven that fear is passed down in the genetic code.

When I speak of using an herbal ally to assist in someone's wellbeing, it is very clear who has remained hostage to this fear. I can identify the fear because I, too, was held hostage to that fear before becoming a mother. My savior was motherhood, experiencing illness within my family and ADHD behavior in the lives of my children. By listening to my own guidance, I knew medications were not the path I wanted to take. This was the beginning of breaking down the walls of fear I once had. In fact, in the 1990s, before the birth of my children, I remember taking antibiotics so I would not get sick with the flu or other supposed sickness. Of course at that time I was sick every few months, had allergies while I also received the flu shot. Believing I was doing everything right, doing what I was "supposed" to do, I was still in the end very weak constitutionally. It is surprising to me as I now understand how devastating antibiotics can be to the immune system, and know they should only be used when all else has not given way to health and vitality.

Over the years, I have thought about this story many times, and tried to imagine a time when our herbal allies were our go-to in wellness. I imagine strong, wise, highly-knowledgeable herbalists, and formulas passed down through the generations. The women drenched in this knowledge would have known the secrets of how to subdue menstrual cramps and birthing pains, or how to release an unwanted pregnancy. The knowledge of which allies to use for natural birth control as well as formulations to use as we age for hormone support into menopause, for both men and women.

I imagine these strong, knowledgeable women being treated unfairly, possibly abused mentally and sexually. I imagine the abuser's intention was to leave this woman with child and also completely dependent upon him. I visualize the anger when he figures out she never becomes pregnant due to the ancient knowledge she holds dear to her. She is able to either release unwanted pregnancies or use her plant allies so to never become pregnant, finding natural birth control time and time again, leaving this woman fully empowered. I then visualize this woman being accused of witchcraft as the abuser turns the townspeople against her with his own need to dominate her. I also imagine these powerful herbalists being feared in their communities due to the uneducated nature of the townspeople. As history has repeated time and time again, mankind will squash and kill when fear is present. This is speculation, as I do not know of such an individual personally, but I feel this vision holds many truths. I believe we have been gifted a medicinal ally for every ailment.

These herbal clinics of the 1800-1900s existed to service the public, and specialized in annual detoxification of the body systems among many other things. The annual clean-out assured health and longevity throughout the year by administering herbal formulations similar to our current day flu shot. The main focus of the herbal clean-out was the elimination of candida or parasites. I would like to highlight the three main herbs as they deserve their time in the spotlight, along with information regarding candida and parasite invasions. My understanding of our herbal allies is that any desired outcome is possible with the correct herbal ally formula and a person who is open to change, holding themselves accountable for the illness, and stepping into their new self.

Candida and parasites can take up permanent living arrangements within our body's systems, wreaking havoc, and are one on the most undiagnosed health threats in the world today. These highlighted herbs are wormwood, black walnut, and clove. I believe these are another example of the holy trinity and become synergistic, vibrational champions when cleaning out unwanted guests.

Parasites include many organisms and are more common than you may think. They are part of a healthy ecosystem. In fact, parasites from tapeworms to candida can become fungal parasites, and have been associated with many disorders ranging from mental confusion and neuron-degeneration to autoimmune diseases like IBS, rheumatoid arthritis, and thyroid disorders. Here is a list of other health disruptions linked to hosting these intruders within our body:

Fatigue   Feeling achy in tendons and muscles
Extreme tightness in shoulder and neck
Acid reflux   Excessive production of mucous
Sleep disturbance   Frequent sore throat
White-coated tongue   Chronic sinus problems
Skin sensitivities— rashes, eczema, dermatitis, acne, dandruff
Skin discolorations   Dental problems
Depression   Irritability
Anxiety / Panic attack / Schizophrenia
Recurring obsessive thoughts
Mood swings   Bad breath
Chills or night sweats   Thyroid imbalance
Shortness of breath   Dizziness - vertigo
Temperature sensitivity   Sweet cravings
Alcohol intolerance   Gluten/casein intolerance
Irregular heartbeat / HBP   IBS - constipation - diarrhea
Gas - abdominal bloating   Dry eyes
Anal discharge or itching   Hormone imbalance
PMS — UTI — Recurrent yeast infections, vaginal or ear infection - thrush

Chronic athletes foot	Toenail/fingernail fungus
Ringing in the ears	Anemia
Allergies to foods - odors - chemicals	
Weight changes without change in diet	
Light-headedness	Foggy thinking
Fainting	Muscle weakness
Restless leg syndrome	Low sex drive
Nausea vomiting	Auto-Immune dysfunction

Weakening of immune system - therefore inviting all disease into the body

Looking at this list it is alarming as these intruders affect every system in our body: circulatory (heart, blood vessels), digestive (stomach, liver, gallbladder, intestines), endocrine (pituitary, thyroid, pancreas, adrenal), integumentary (hair, skin, nails), skeletal system (cartilage, bones, joints) lymphatic (thymus, nodes, spleen), respiratory (nasal, trachea, lungs), muscular (muscles, tendons), nervous (brain, spinal cord, nerves), renal / urinary systems (kidneys, bladder) and reproductive system.

This is not to say that if you have many of the above symptoms, you are riddled with invaders. But I would like to point out that using the holy trinity of herbs is highly affordable, non-toxic (also given to my canine BFF), vibrationally healing, incredibly nutrient-dense and have many other health benefits I will outline below. Why not consider an annual clean out or just bring these allies into your lifestyle?

When living in an industrialized country, you may think parasites are horror stories from developing countries, or that the closest you would come to a parasitic infection is traveler's diarrhea. In the U.S. you can pick up a parasite from a restaurant or tick / insect bite from your family pet, etc.

Other ways to acquire a parasite/candida include:

unwashed fruits and veggies
eating sushi
kissing a pet, cuddling a pet
sharing a couch or bed with your pet
drinking tap water or well-water
sex / kissing with a person hosting the intruders
passing the intruders to our unborn babies

These unwelcome guests are actually a sign of an intact, unstressed ecosystem, and the opposite, as strange as it may sound, is true: if parasites / candida disappear from our environment, the habitat probably is in trouble. Bugs, whether bacteria, viruses, fungi, and even larger, creepy crawly critters, are naturally part of our world.

The traditional western lifestyle is set to leave us vulnerable with internal weakness and imbalance, making these intruders more problematic. These unwelcome guests have an intricate form of self-defense: they are immune to antibiotics and able to build a wall of mucus as defense (biofilm). Chemo or radiation would be the most potent form of protection to cast the unwelcome from the body, in the traditional lifestyle setting.

A parasite clean-out removes these unwelcome guests as well as common pathogenic bugs and keeps our body systems unburdened. These unwelcome guests set off massive amounts of inflammation throughout all of our body's systems, ending in our GI tract. Inflammation creates permeability, when the walls of the gut and GI become inflamed and permeable, any pathogen can enter the bloodstream. Inflammation will effect all areas of the body as well, from arthritis to HPB and cancer. Inflammation is the butterfly effect catalyst. Inflammation of the GI tract will eventually lead to inflammation of the brain, giving host to an array of mental challenges. Inflammation of the joints will eventually lead to bone and tissue lose. The butterfly effect means that when seemingly insignificant changes are made, the results can have a major impact. For instance, by reducing the inflammation of the GI tract, one may feel vibrant, clear-headed, and all-around happy. It is said in alternative wellness that when the GI tract is inflamed, the mind is confused and toxic, as there is an energetic connection between the two, just as there is a connection to the toxicity of the lungs and the health of fine china.

Candida is a plant-like fungus that begins its life as yeast. Not all candida or yeast are considered unfavorable or bad for the body, but it can become overgrown and take your body hostage. Candida and parasites travel together like twins that never separate. If the nutritional intake of the host is nurturing for the unwelcome guests, combined with slow digestion, which is currently the digestive health of most of the U.S., then we become the most nurturing host. With a sluggish digestive tract, the chosen standard American diet sits in the GI tract, fermenting alcohol and toxins that kill the "good" bacteria. Without good bacteria our unwelcome guests grow at exponential rates.

The "good" bacteria have many benefits throughout our body systems. One amazing benefit is regulating the t-cell function (immune system). As their population declines, so does the immune system.

Candida eats by injecting the surrounding area with exo-enzymes, dissolving it so the roots can suck up the nutrients. As the unwelcome guests feast, they release mycotoxins or poisons, giving the body symptoms of infection and inflammation, such as IBS, irregular bowel movements, arthritis, and digestive issues. Candida will shift into the mycelial form, sending roots like hyphae for duplication. When two roots meet they can split one of their cells and combine to form a new cell or spore, and so on and so forth, ensuring their survival. You get the picture: they are gross, colonized, and powerful.

Upon colonization of the host, these unwelcome guests create a barrier called a biofilm. Biofilm forms a layer of protection around the entire colony of unwelcome guests. The biofilm is made of very, very tacky or gummy mucus. I was fortunate to experience the elimination of biofilm within my own body, as it came up through my lungs and out my GI tract during my 3rd or 4th clean-out. It was the strangest, grossest, tackiest substance I've ever seen leave my body, and I'm a mother of two beauties. After the release of this biofilm, my allergies and mucus congestion within my lungs completely disappeared. Many organisms will embed themselves into this biofilm for protection. The biofilm is a barrier that will protect the bad microorganisms from our immune system. This biofilm also assists the intruders, evading the effects of anti-parasitic substances, i.e., probiotics or antibiotics (traditional therapies do not have a remedy or a conclusive test).

However, when using our amazing plant allies, the biofilm is destroyed and cast from the body. The saying "don't mess with mother nature" fits well here. This happens all while leaving the beneficial flora (the good guys, probiotics) intact and unharmed. I imagine the probiotics I consume during a clean out, finding the holy trinity plant allies within the body, and singing hallelujah, joining forces, and dominantly expelling the unwelcome guests. The plant kingdom has shown itself to work synergistically and vibrantly since the beginning of herbalism, thousands of years ago, to assist mankind in every way possible. We are truly here to help one another.

The probiotic or good bacteria can also create their own healthy biofilm, which can actually help heal inflammation throughout our body systems.

When a person's body is a gracious host for unwelcome guests, there is a correlation with high levels of mercury, lead, iron, and fluoride. These metals and toxins assist in hosting mainly as a method of transportation, as candida and parasites can attach to these molecules and travel throughout your body. The general consensus is that yeast is an immune response to mercury / parasite poisoning. With thyroid imbalance the link to metals and other toxins are commonly found.

In my opinion, the unwelcome guest clean-out process is the very basis for all bodies seeking optimum health. This is the foundation for all operating systems of the body to function at their highest frequency: vibrant, alert, and eager for life's journey, whatever that may be. When looking at the journey of the clean-out process, it can be difficult, especially for first or second-time participants. When these unwelcome guests are evicted or die, they release toxic gases and waste (the liver eliminates it), which can make you feel horrible, like you have the flu, but only for a short while. When the body has been completely invaded by the intruders, it is all the more necessary to take the journey for optimum health and happiness. This reaction is called "die-off symptoms" it is an unfortunate part of the clean-out process. It is essential to give yourself space for this journey to release, shift, heal, and transform. I recommend when you venture on your first journey, begin slowly and reduce the dosage for a few weeks, allowing the liver to properly keep up with the toxins emitted from the die-off symptoms. This is the time for you to listen to your body, to follow what it asks you to do. There is no need to be over aggressive and start with the maximum suggested dosage as odds are you will feel horrible and quit. This is another opportunity to step into the vibration of "To become your own healer, you need only listen to your inner-voice."

During the clean out, nutritional intake is very important for prompt, proper elimination. It is recommended to consume probiotics and a bowel cleanser (herbal) during this process. Be sure to take these supplements individually, as you want complete control over how many capsules your body may need for a bowel-clean out. Some people may need one a day and some may need five a day, but you do not want the holy trinity mixed with the bowel-cleaning herbs. Take them separately. After completion of the clean-out phase, the next step is to remove metals and tone the organs. This is all accomplished with our herbal allies, and during this stage you will feel amazing.

It is recommended to repeat the clean-out six months later, and then annually thereafter. But my body tells me gently to journey every 6 to 7 months. After the die-off symptoms subside, I love the way I feel and so does my body. But it took a few clean-out journeys to have little to no die-off symptoms. Whether it is your first journey or fourth one (after the die-off symptoms pass) you can expect to feel energetic, clear-headed, allergy free, with smooth and glowing skin, free of body odor or with less odor for some, and your eyesight may even improve. As you can see, my body loves the holy trinity, but it was a process to arrive here.

I attempted to rid my body of these invaders after a detoxification class in 2008. This instructor showed pictures of different parasites and worms, which was disgusting. I really wanted them out of my body, so I tried to "tough it out" with a dosage that was too high for my level of invasion. It made for a difficult journey. The reality is I did not listen to the guidance of my own body, and allowed my mind to take over. Just relax and trust.

The journey of the clean out is a process that takes time, depending on one's level of infestation. It is not possible to be free of these invaders for long, as they are part of our environment. The clean out is to keep them at a manageable level, and to keep ourselves at optimum performance, similar to the never ending process of exterminating your house for termites. The holy trinity of herbal allies has alternative beneficial actions beyond the clean out. These herbs are part of complete well-being. Truthfully, my body was completely invaded with unwelcome guests and was not able to process the release of toxins quickly enough to maintain a feeling of wellness. I urge you to listen to your body, as it truly knows what is best for itself. Take it slow with minimum dosage, breathe a lot (70% of toxic waste is in the breath), and the remainder is within urination, bowel, and body secretions. You can do simple things during the transition, i.e., salt baths, body brushing, stretching (yoga), massage, reiki treatment, and meditation.

When the body is free from stress or the fight or flight response, it allows for a state of relaxation, and this is the only state the body is able to heal itself.

HOLY TRINITY:

Here is a deeper look into the benefits of the holy trinity of herbal allies: cloves, wormwood, and black walnut. If you are pregnant, nursing, or taking any medications, always consult your doctor and a certified herbalist before consuming any herbal ally new to your body systems.

Cloves - (Syzygium aromaticum)
Will smooth and relax intestines/GI tract, aid in digestion/gas, increase metabolism, reduce stomach ache, vomiting, diarrhea, expectorant of phlegm, reduce tooth pain, sun burn, arthritis, poison ivy, sinusitis, antimicrobial, kill parasites and bad bacteria in GI tract, relieve excess bloating, gas, morning sickness, anti-histamine, anti-inflammatory, enhance sexual health (aphrodisiac), protect liver, fight cancer (used in lung cancer), boost the immune system, control diabetes, used for tooth decay, bad breath, anti-oxidant, preserve bone density, relieve headaches, remove acne, clear blemishes and scars, relieve anxiety, and prevent hair loss.

Wormwood - (Artemisia absinthium)
Considered a bitter and used in absinthe, vermouth and bitters. Stimulates GI and gallbladder function, liver support, produces bile to aid gallbladder, expelling of intestinal worms, kills malaria, kills cancer cells, anti-microbial and anti-fungal, anti-bacteria, aids with insomnia, stimulates menstruation to assist with irregular periods, stimulates cerebral hemispheres and balances grey matter, aids in neurasthenia (helps to cure mental illness, schizophrenia), muscle relaxant, brings childbirth and afterbirth, anti-anxiety, mild sedative, stimulates poor circulation, balances appetite (anorexia, over eating), cleans internal organs, positive effects on Crohn's disease and any other disease pertaining the digestive tract, anti-oxidant, and revitalizes enzyme production.

Black Walnut - (Juglans Nigra)

Antibacterial, anti-cancer, anti-diarrheic, anti-hepatoxic (prevents damage to the liver), chelator, anti-hypertensive, anti-tumor, anti-ulcer, anti-fungal, externally used for jock itch, dermatitis, ringworm, athlete's foot, blisters, scabbing pruritus, varicose ulcers and syphilis sores, leprosy and gangrene. Use to expel worms, parasites, candida and harmful pathogens from the body. Alter the ph of the intestines, which helps kill fungus, parasites, yeast and expels all toxins. Also useful for cell damage caused by liver injury due to exposure to certain toxins, supports thyroid and metabolism (iodine), normalizes blood sugar, cardiovascular and cholesterol control, supports weight loss, assists with acne, eczema, and psoriasis, wards off warts, cold sores, and herpes, reduces excessive sweating, anti-inflammatory for digestive tract, treats both constipation and diarrhea, and is a sore throat treatment.

Wow, right? They are amazing, and I am only skimming the surface of the medicinal qualities in these allies. These allies assist each of our body's systems, including reproductive health. My intention is to share knowledge and connect to Gaia in a way that opens doorways to individual research, as each medicinal ally has it own relationship to each individual, and will show up as needed in your life. Just open your front door and discover the gifts Gaia has sent to you. My favorite brands for the clean-out are scram, parasitin, or para-smart.

Returning to the story shared by my instructor, can you see how these herbal clinics of long ago may have once been a threat to big business pharmacy? If one chose to clean and clear their body systems and reduce the threat of disease, then how would a system built mainly on symptom relief stand to make a profit?

"The most effective way to do it, is to do it."
-Amelia Earhart

FINE CHINA SUPPOSITORY FORMULA

Let's return the focus to the herbal allies in the fine china suppository formula. I used many herbal allies, feeling each ally had their own role to play, and needed the support of neighboring allies to have the power to lift mind/ body/ spirit to optimum health. One of my favorite herbal allies is astragalus. I want to scream "Wow!" or should I say "Will you allow me to wow you with its amazingness?" My first introduction to astragalus was back in 2001, when my son was just 2 years old. The study of the healing arts was not on the horizon, and he had a serious sinus infection. I was at work, speaking with my pediatrician's office on the phone, and the nurse recommended another prescription for his third round of antibiotics. I responded with: "If two rounds have not given him relief, why would you think a third round would?" I felt confused as I wanted to trust the recommendation, but my body was telling me it was not right. I felt confused after hanging up the phone. I did not have the experience or knowledge to help him. Lucky for me, one of my coworkers overheard the conversation. This beauty was originally from South Africa, had her own natural healing story of healing stomach cancer, and was wise and knowledgeable. She informed me that when children from her country have ear or sinus infections, they do not treat it with antibiotics. Strange, I thought, because that is the only way we treat these infections in this country. I asked "What do you do?" She said "We use tinctures of astragalus and eyebright." At that moment in my life those herbs may as well have been a foreign language. Really, they were a foreign language.

I felt hopeful with the recommendation and promptly purchased the tincture. Within one day I noticed a shift in him, and on the second day their was noticeable improvement in his breathing, and the mucus began to thin and clear. I was deeply grateful for her wisdom, and astounded with the results. It appears clear to me as I write these words that I listened to my body signals when dealing with those I hold dear to me better than listening to my body signals when dealing with myself. Of course, this was 2001, and I was diagnosed in 2015, so I am grateful I finally absorbed the life lesson.

I believe astragalus deserves a proper introduction, I want to include a research paper I wrote during the Essential Application of Herbology Course. I've revised it a little and thoroughly enjoyed digging deep into the this highly medicinal herbal ally. I hope you enjoy it as well.

Astragalus Membranaceous:

The root is used and is harvested at approximately four years old. This herbal ally has been used in traditional Chinese medicine (TCM) for thousands of years. Astragalus is easily combined with other herbs to strengthen the body against disease. TCM used it for autoimmune disorders, to normalize and balance the immune system (in the US we caution for autoimmune or overstimulation of the immune system). It also promotes phagocytosis (swallows up foreign cells or particles by immune system cells).

In Japan, a study from School of Medicine showed it increased B cells production (which produce antibody, and seek and destroy invaders) and increased T cells (white blood cells, which find and destroy invaders), increased interleukin and antibody production, increased leukocytes (hunter t cells to help to identify viruses, bacteria, and other rouge cells, and destroy them). Astragalus increases the production of our killer hunter cells, then empowers the body to do what it needs to in order to find optimum health and vitality. Amazing!

In the US, we are looking to use it as a treatment for people whose immune system is weak from chemo or radiation due to the decline in white blood cell count. When the count goes too low, the therapy must stop because the patient is high risk for infections, thus giving cancer a chance to regenerate. Astragalus helps to feed the white blood cells and continue therapy. Studies have shown patients recovered faster and lived longer when taking astragalus.

Astragalus acts through the same pathways that are the target of many chemotherapy drugs, including PARP inhibition and inhibition of the P13K-Akt pathway that are so common in many women's cancers.

This next part is absolutely mind-blowing, or so I would think if the above hadn't blown it away already. I hope to explain this in a way that does justice, as some of the terminology is difficult to relay.

Amazing astragalus is also able to activate a key enzyme called telomerase. This enzyme promotes the production of telomeres: tell=end, meros=part.

Telomeres are attached to the end part of our DNA chromosomes, and help keep the DNA together during the replication process. They act like the plastic end-caps of shoelaces, preventing the lace from fraying and being damaged.

Each time a cell is replicated it is shortened, however, with telomeres protecting the ends (providing we have enough telomeres), the only part of the chromosome that is lost is the telomere, and the DNA is left undamaged. Without telomeres, important DNA would be lost every time a cell divides, and would lead to loss of the entire gene and cell death.

With cell death you have aging/premature aging and onset of disease and death. Astragalus again feeds the enzyme telomerase to assist in production and abundance of telomeres. Assuring the abundance of telomeres for DNA protection during replication and longevity of the chromosome induces youthful vitality.

There are many main components but the polysaccharides (*long chain of sugar molecules, anti-obesity, anti-diabetic, anti-carcinogenic, anti-microbial, anti-viral, anti-tumor, anti-inflammatory, immune building, prebiotic for digestive system*), the same as in shiitake mushrooms, a favorite in the macrobiotic lifestyle, are known to "seek and destroy cancer cells."

A Chinese herbalist, Li Ching-yun, supposedly lived to be over 256 years old. The Chinese government congratulated him on his 150th and 200th birthdays, as reported by the New York Times in 1933. This story is inspiring, with some disagreements on his age at death. He did survive quite a few wives. Give or take a few decades, this man lived beyond the years of any other known human being. Salute to Gaia and all her beauty and may Li Ching-yun rest in peace.

Astragalus is used for:

Slows signs of aging	Anemia
Diuretic - clears edema	Increases endurance
Vasodilator	Lowers blood pressure
Improves liver function	Candida control
Aids digestion	Anti-inflammatory
Colds & flu, influenza	Herpes
Diabetes - regulates blood sugar	Mono / assists during chemo
Chronic fatigue syndrome	Lack of appetite from chemo
Heart disease	Hypoglycemia
Hepatitis	Kidney & liver disease
Fibromyalgia	Seasonal allergies

Treats prolapsed organs especially the uterus
Uterine bleeding after childbirth
Cancer - bone, breast, cervical, vaginal, colorectal, endometrial, Hodgkins, kidney, liver, lung, ovarian

Burns & abbesses - topically	Anti-bacterial, antimicrobial, antiviral
Modulates overactive immune system	Anti-hepatotoxic (nourishes the liver)

Adaptogen - protects body against various stresses physical/mental/emotional

Cardio protective	Elevates mood

Form of usage:

Tincture   Capsules   Topically for skin
Injectable form in Asian countries   soups or broths and teas

Children:

yes

Adult dosage:

Tea 9-15 grams day   capsules 250-500mg 3x day
Can be taken tonically / long term

Great for our Canine BFFs

No known side effects

No evidence if safe for pregnant or breastfeeding mothers
Caution in the U.S. for autoimmune disease

Drug Interactions:
Any drug that suppresses the immune system
cyclophosphamide (med used to reduce chances of transplant
rejection)
corticosteroids
lithium

Astragalus is one of my first loves. Did you say "wow" to
any of the above? I hope this ally ignites your passion for seeking
more information, as there is always a deeper layer in the study of
herbology.

This herbal ally was part of my morning tea, herbal supplements,
and vaginal suppository formula through the healing phase of

my vaginal cancer, as well as taken tonically over a few months. Astragalus can easily become part of your garden, as it grows easily in the USA, and would love to be part of your life.

Yellow Dock - (Rumex crispus)

The next champion ally of my vaginal formula which deserves our attention and adoration is yellow dock.

I also wrote a research paper on this ally for my Plant Connection course. I again was completely blown away with its medicinal properties. This ally is part of the California School of Herbal Studies (CSHS) list of top 30 herbs. Yellow dock is also in the Essaic formula, which is responsible for assisting thousands of people with healing cancer and other degenerative diseases. Although the Essiac formula had been used by the Canadian Indians eons before its release, this formula was introduced in the 1930s and brought into our world by Renee Caisse. If you have not read her story, I encourage you to, it is inspiring! Her book is "Calling of an Angel" The True Story of Rene Caisse and an Indian Herbal Medicine Called Essiac, Nature's Cure for Cancer. Blessings to Rene Caisse and may she rest in peace.

I did not use the Essiac formula specifically for the healing of my cancer, but I have used it with my mother. She's 79 years young and a rock star: 64 year smoker, spots on her lungs, COPD, pneumonia frequently. She has taken Essiac for about 3 months, and has been feeling amazing. At her recent doctor's appointment for her liver (she has degenerative disease, from statins years ago, and smoking), her doctor was astonished at how wonderful her blood work and ultrasound of her liver appeared. Of course, I cannot leave out that she stopped smoking, and I am so proud of Mama. The best news I could have asked for. Now, if I can just get her to believe Gaia has herbal allies specifically for liver rejuvenation, clearing cirrhosis and other disease, and returning vitality to this very important organ. Baby steps. One thing I have learned in becoming an herbalist is to allow clients to process in their own time. The saying "When the student is ready, the teacher appears," fits perfectly here.

Yellow Dock – Greek, means "to cleanse"
also known as - sheep sorrel, curled dock, narrow dock, sorrel

Botanical Name
Rumex Crispus

Family
Polygonaceae

Grows in a variety of habitats, from open fields to transition areas with direct or partial sunlight, prefers high acidity soil, slightly elevated, slightly moist soils, but can tolerate dry rocky or sandy soil. Has been considered a nuisance and pesky weed. Grows as a taproot about 2 to 3 feet deep, and spreads laterally to a radius of 8 to 12 inches. In larger areas with sandy soil, it can grow larger, and if grown in clay soil the radius is smaller. The roots are harvested after the plant has died back, and the best roots are 3 to 4 years old. All parts of the plant can be used and eaten. It is a perennial with drooping pale green or red flowers that turn to rusty brown. It will grow from 1 to 3 feet high. The leaves are most tasty when young and have a lemony flavor. Steam and serve with garlic and olive oil (more carotene than carrots). Flowering season is June to July. To home garden, it must have a deep porous garden bed.

Constituents: magnesium, oxalic acid, selenium, silicon, sodium, tannis, iron, phosphorus, calcium, vitamin A and C, (when combined with dandelion and nettle, is a treatment for anemia), rumicin is an active compound in the root, contains chrysarobin - used to treat skin conditions as well as a congested liver.

History: In North America, from the beginning, and from 1700-1900, it was used as a pot herb by the settlers. The leaves were boiled in lard or sweet cream for ulcers / sore eyes / glandular swelling. The roots and seeds were given in cases of dysentary. Before the settlers, the Indians used it as medicine and also yellow dye. The bruised root was used as a poultice for abrasions, sores, itchy skin, and eruptions.

In 1653, Nicholas Culpepper was quoted as saying: "All Docks are under Jupiter, of which the Red Dock, which is commonly called Bloodwort - cleanses the blood and strengthens the liver. But, Yellow Dock Root is best taken when either the blood or liver is affected by Choler. All have cooling, drying qualities. Yellow Dock being most cool and Bloodwort most drying."

Researchers in Akilu Emma Institute of Pathobiology in Ethiopia conducted a study to estimate healing properties of therapeutic plants. Yellow dock root scored among the highest for its detoxifying and antioxidant properties.

In a study in 2012, it displayed "remarkable cytotoxic activities" on several tested leukemia cell lines, meaning it has the ability to kill and destroy cancer cells.

Yellow Dock is used for -

Anemia	Blood cleanser/lymph cleanser
Pain and swelling of nasal and respiratory passages	
Bacterial infections	S.T.D.s & U.T.I.s
Scurvy	Diarrhea & constipation
Heavy menstrual bleeding	Laxative
Jaundice	Antioxidant
Anti-cancer	Skin tonic
Depurative (purifying)	Cholagague (stimulates bile)
Anorexia	Reduces inflammation
Gastritis	Colitis
I.B.S.	Swollen lymph glands
Mouth ulcers	Fibrocystic breasts
Uterine fibroids & tumors	Acne / boils / eczema

Rheumatoid arthritis   Gout

Fibromyalgia

Aids liver & gallbladder, aids in low stomach acid. Stimulates production of bile to aid digestion. Stimulates bowel movement, removes lingering waste from intestine, and aids urine to release toxins from tissues. Supports lymphatic and blood circulation, liver, colon, and kidney function.

James Green, master herbalist & author of The Herbal Medicine-Makers Handbook, states "yellow dock is a wonderful alternative for treating oily and oxidative skin conditions. It seems to work through the liver and bowel to help remove metabolic wastes from the blood. By improving the liver's ability to metabolize wastes and fats, it takes the burden off of secondary pathways of eliminations, such as the skin."

On the List of 30 Top Herbs for California School of Herbal Studies CSHS.

Dosage - non-toxic and can be combined with other herbs 20-25% of formulation. Best herbs to blend with: burdock, cleavers, yellow bedstraw, elecampane root, sweet clover, dandelion root-leaf-flower, red clover flower, stinging nettle, blue violet, and hibiscus.

In the U.S., a "warning" for oxalates, as may cause kidney damage (this in extremely high dosage) and not recommended during pregnancy. However, In Harmony Herbs in Ocean Beach, San Diego has yellow dock in a pregnancy tea formula: red raspberry leaf, chamomile, yellow dock root, dandelion leaf, nettles, peppermint, rosehips. Delicious, and I drink even though I am not expecting, as this formula is highly nutritive and supportive for all body systems. I find most "warnings" are from studies of an isolated compound of the plant and dosage is also extremely high. While consuming the whole plant the magical buffers given by Gaia are of most importance and will keep the body systems in balance.

Interactions:

Digoxin - Lanoxin (lower potassium levels), and water pills (diuretic drugs)
Moderate interaction with Warfarin (coumadin)
Tea - straight up it is strong, bitter, and dry. For class demonstrations I blend yellow dock with burdock and vanilla.

Yellow Dock Tea -

6 cups of un-fluorinated, filtered water
3t yellow dock root
2t burdock (optional) or other herb
1t real organic vanilla extract
raw honey or natural sweetener to taste

Boil, low, add 4 cups water with herbs for 15 minutes, covered
Turn off heat, cool add vanilla
Brew 30 - 60 minutes if desired
Add 2 cups of water, reheat, and serve
Pour through a strainer. Add honey or stevia to taste.

In the Essiac formula, the herb is left to brew for 12 or more hours for cancer treatment medicine. This form of brewing is a decoction and is very strong medicine.

Thank you for your time and hope this project opened doors for the many uses of this amazing plant. Blessings.

Reference list:

Anniesremedy.com
globalhealingctr.com
webmd.com
Story of Rene Caisse

The Herbal Medicine-Makers Handbook, James Green

That completes the sharing of my research paper. I hope learning about yellow dock has awoken your inner desire for more knowledge. This paper just skimmed the surface of what yellow dock is capable of. I love this champion.

Echinacea - (Echinacea Purpurea)

The next herbal ally within the fine china suppository is echinacea, most beloved herb of America. It was originally used by our Native Americans for snake bite, colic, and infection. The ally boosts immune system, encourages healthy cell growth, increases oxygen in the blood, reduces anxiety, depression, aches and pains, improves insulin resistance in diabetes, supports the respiratory system, is anti-aging, anti-cancer, anti microbial, anti-viral, anti-oxidant, and anti inflammatory.

Cheers to echinacea.

The next herbal ally champion I would like to introduce is poke root. This herbal ally was new to me prior to my diagnosis, but, its medicinal qualities deserve a proper introduction.

Poke Root - (Phytolacca Americana)

Poke root dates back before the settlers and was used in America by the Native Americans. This herb is known for its use with the upper respiratory tract and lymphatic congestion. It has been used for tonsillitis, catarrh, laryngitis, swollen glands, breasts, throat, groin, mastitis, mumps, acne, boils, degenerative gum disease, herpes, chicken pox, shingles, tumors, impetigo, ringworm, hemorrhoids, headaches, swelling of sprains, as a spermicide, immune builder (enhance T-cell count), anti-inflammatory, anti-viral (HIV, HPV, herpes, poliovirus, influenza), detoxing effect on organs and revitalizes their efficiency, gonorrhea, syphilis, rheumatism eruptions, cancers: vaginal/liver /blood, stimulates spleen function, reduces inflammation of spleen, endometriosis, and headaches.

One of my favorite tinctures from Wishgarden herbs is Kick-Ass Sinus, and poke root is one of the ingredients. Poke root is valued within the tincture for its specific job: poking at inflamed tissue. This is valuable because toxins become stuck in areas of inflammation, which increases the inflammation, making the tissue more uncomfortable and unable to heal. When poke root arrives at the area of inflammation it "pokes" at the inflamed tissue, thus allowing the tissue to ooze and release, giving way to toxin removal and reducing inflammation. How incredible of a job does poke root have, and how lucky are we to know such an ally?

Poke root, taken in large doses, can be a powerful emetic (vomiting) and purgative (diarrhea) and should be used in a highly respectful nature.

It is recommended as a blended herb in herbal formulations or as a tea (1/4 teaspoon in a cup of hot water) a few times a day.

Poke root is mind-blowingly amazing, wouldn't you say?

The next herbal ally champion within the suppository that I would like to introduce is goldenseal root.

Goldenseal root - (Hydrastis canadensis)

This plant is an at-risk plant (has not been properly wildcrafted, has been over-used, and is endangered). Use only cultivated plants, or use barberry or Oregon grape, as they have similar actions.

Goldenseal is one of the California School of Herbal Studies top 30 herbal allies.

Goldenseal root and rhizome are mostly used medicinally, have been used in history for many aliments, and date back to before the settlers. Goldenseal is a bitter, so it is a digestive stimulant, hepatic (detoxifies and tones the liver), cholagogue (promotes flow of bile from gallbladder), antimicrobial, antibiotic, anti-inflammatory, anti-cancer, anti-catarrhal (used with sinus infections), respiratory system to balance and tone mucous membranes, urinary system (UTI), astringent (firms and strengthens body tissues), skin disorders (eczema, ringworm, puritis, conjunctivitis, gums ulcer, thrush), fever reducer, relieves congestion (whooping cough), pneumonia, colitis, dyspepsia, reduces cholesterol, used during labor to bring contractions, destroys protozoa, fungi, streptococci, diarrhea, E.Coli, salmonella, giardia, cholera, and candida. As a circulatory herb it enhances heart function and stimulates the immune system and the production of white blood cells.

Goldenseal is not recommended during pregnancy as it can stimulate the involuntary muscles of the uterus.

This herbal ally is just amazing and I hope you found it to be as well.

This next herbal ally champion included within the suppository is tea tree oil and most definitely deserves a proper introduction. The formula I used for my vaginal suppository called for just a few drops of this very potent ally. The essential oil is the most powerful of all herbal medicines and should be used graciously, with purpose and restraint.

Tea Tree Oil - (Melaleuca Alternifolia)

Melaleuca alternifolia is the same plant manuka honey is made from. Melaleuca's origins go back to New Zealand, although California's central valley is looking to become a producer of the shrub, but will probably genetically modify it as most plants in the valley are GMO. New Zealand is known for organic farming practices and I personally look for melaleuca of New Zealand origin.

Tea tree oil has been used for aromatherapy (raising our vibration, receiving healing properties), lung spa (steaming lungs, breathing), athletes foot, dandruff, acne, ringworm, candida/yeast infection, lice, nail fungus, herpes, insect repellant, scabies, eczema, psoriasis, skin abrasions, sore throat, kills protozoa, expectorant, boosts the immune system, relieves muscle pains & strains, oral health (bleeding gums, tooth decay, kills halitosis), eliminates body odor by destroying bacteria-producing odor, ear infections, anti-microbial, and anti-fungal.

Tea tree oil is not recommended during pregnancy or taken internally. When used on the skin, a carrier oil should be used.

I hope you said wow at least one time.

Turmeric - (Curcuma longa)

This next herbal ally champion is turmeric. This brilliantly-colored cooking spice has recently begun to have its day of notoriety. This herb most definitely deserves a proper introduction. Although turmeric has been in use for years, it is only recently that the USA has enjoyed its culinary and medical properties. Turmeric's origin is from South Asia, used as a culinary spice in curry and used in the goldenmilk recipe and within the suppository formula.

Turmeric has been used for anti-aging, arthritis, anti-inflammatory (eases joint-pain), anti-oxidant, anti-microbial (acne), reduces free radical damage, Crohn's, protects the heart, lowers the risk of heart disease (needs black pepper or cayenne pepper for maximum absorption potential), antibiotic, anti-obesity, anti-cancer (destroys cancer cells), fights diabetes, colitis, heals gut, IBS, gas, bloating, gallbladder disorder, high cholesterol, fatigue, assists long-term memory, protects from depression, regulates neurotransmitters (serotonin and dopamine), treats Alzheimer's, protects the brain during the aging process. In China it is used to treat early stages of cervical cancer.

Can be used topically (vaginal formula) or internally (golden milk recipe & curry).

Curcumin is part of turmeric, and for my healing, I used the whole plant turmeric (root). I believe when medicinal components are taken out of their natural habitat and isolated, they are no longer in balance, but I realize many receive benefit from curcumin.

Turmeric is likely safe in the amounts used in cooking, so make this amazing herbal ally part of your daily diet. During pregnancy, turmeric is likely safe when used as a spice in the daily diet, but taken medically, it may stimulate the uterus.

Caution for those with gallbladder problems, as it may slow blood clotting, diabetes, and GERD when taken medically or in capsule form. Also caution for those with vaginal or breast cancers as turmeric can assist in the production of estrogen, however, turmeric is used to assist in healing these cancers as well. What I have found when cautions appear, is that often the plant has been used at an exceptionally high dose and isolated components of the plant are used, therefore losing the magical buffers mother nature has provided for maintaining balance within the body systems.

Cayenne Pepper - (Capsicum annuum)

This last herbal ally champion really needs no introduction. When this vibrant pepper is in the vicinity you can smell its fragrant sent, it may burn if you hold it in your fingers, and your eyes may even begin to tear. This champion in none other than cayenne pepper. The suppository called for just a touch, but wow!, I was able to feel its potency during treatment, without a doubt. Its main duty is to increase circulation (aid the cardiovascular system while moving bad bacteria and toxins out of the body). It will also increase the potency of the other herbal allies, allowing their strengths to be at the highest vibration. This ally is also known for strengthening the heart, arteries, capillaries, blood flow, nerves and able to clear clogged arteries. It aids the digestive system and immune system, keeping colds and catarrh away. It has been known to eliminate acidity, regulate blood sugar, relieve hemorrhoids, ulcers, and heartburn. Used topically, it will warm the hands and feet. This ally is also known to help with delirium, tremors, gout, paralysis, fever, dyspepsia, flatulence, sore throat, menorrhagia, coughs, diarrhea, and it's a carminative and sialagogue (promotes saliva).

Binding Agent

The vaginal suppository had a binding agent, as something was needed to hold the team together. When choosing an ally for such a job, one must use a product free from anything artificial - petroleum, parabens, or fragrance. I used organic coconut oil (OCO) for this very important role.

I'm sure most of you have already heard some of the amazing benefits of OCO, as it has become very popular. This ally can be used for almost everything and deserves a proper introduction. For starters, it is wonderful to cook with and is able to handle high temperatures before oxidation can begin or transition to a carcinogenic level.

OCO can be added to smoothies, morning porridge, used for oral hygiene by holding a dollop of oil for 10-20 minutes a few times a week, your mouth, gums and teeth will thank you as it can reduce gingivitis, inflammation, halitosis, reduce headaches and improve the function of the immune system. OCO is anti-viral and anti-microbial and is also able to whiten teeth. It has be used to regulate metabolism, support the immune system, healthy fat for the heart, bring energy to a tired body, the auric acid with the oil is second to breastmilk, brings mood balance; reduce anxiety and depression and support thyroid. Has been used to treat influenza, herpes, cancer, measles, hepatitis, SARA, UTI, pneumonia, gonorrhea, measles, improve sleep, balance glucose, diabetes, hemorrhoids, destroy candida/parasites, dissolve kidney stones, promotes natural hormone production, increase absorption of cal/mag, reduce osteoporosis, prevent liver disease, kidney disease/ pancreas / gall bladder disease, prevent atherosclerosis, diaper rash, athletes foot and ringworm.

Topically OCO has been know for use on hair, skin and nails. OCO is moisturizing and promotes elasticity, promotes cell regeneration, and reduces cellulite when used long term.

Each Herbal Ally in the suppository formula is just Amazing, would you agree? This part of the suppository would increase or decrease my frequency? Undeniable increase my vibration.

This suppository is the meaning of living, vibrational medicine. The fine china suppository was used for 5 to 7 days, I felt my skin lesions vanish by 2nd day but continued to day 6.

Each ally was chopped finely, the roots are most difficult and should be ground individually. A coffee grinder is great for this job.

Please seek professional advise.

"The question isn't who's going to let me; it's who's going to stop me.

Ayn Rand

PRE-SUPPOSITORY

Garlic - (Allium sativum)

Prior to using the herbal suppository described above, there was also a period of pre-suppository, or prepping the fine china by moving out old stagnant unwelcome visitors. The powerful pre-suppository is simply an organic garlic clove. This ally was inserted just past the pubic bone for 5 to 7 days. Some prefer to thread a string through the clove before insertion, but I did not and found the clove easy to remove. My treatment lasted 5 days, and I also treated the colon by inserting a sliver of garlic for the same time period. The clove was left in overnight. In the morning, I removed the clove, douched with distilled water and organic apple cider vinegar, then allowed my body to rest for the day before repeating in the evening.

If you are someone who cannot tolerate garlic in your food, especially raw garlic, know that your digestive disputes can mean the garlic is killing off unwelcome guests (candida, worms, parasites), causing die-off symptoms within the gut. Basically, the need for the holy trinity of herbs is a must, and should be part of your near future to ensure a complete cleanup and restoration of the body systems.

Garlic is another true champion for mankind, known to stop the big, bad biofilm from taking over the body's systems. Garlic is used to kill off many of the different strains of candida, as well as killing off parasites, worms, and other unwelcome guests. This very intelligent ally does this without killing off our beneficial bacteria. How does this ally know beneficials from unwelcome guests? Science is just beginning to understand this synergistic flow of Gaia. In fact, I recently listened to a Ted Talk on the underground energetic connections in our forests, and science proven communication exists from plant to plant. One detail I found comforting is when a sapling is just beginning its life, nearby full-grown giants will send nutrients to the baby tree to ensure its strength and ability to grow. Giving and generosity are abundant in nature when we take time to notice.

Does that warm your heart? It really did mine. Avatar is not so far from the truth.

Other uses of our champion garlic include treatment of fungal infections of the skin, the digestive system, vaginal and reproduction system, and for earaches or ear infections by placing a sliver of juicy garlic in a tissue at the opening of the ear, or making a liquid of distilled water and garlic juice to use as an ear wash. Finish the treatment with a swish of organic apple cider vinegar to ensure the quick population of beneficial bacteria. Garlic is known to combat the common cold and flu, reduce blood pressure and regulate blood sugar / diabetes, improve cholesterol, lower risk of heart disease, stroke, cancer, and infections. It may prevent Alzheimer's and dementia, also known to improve athletic performance, aid in detox of heavy metals, and improve bone health. Lastly, garlic is antibacterial and antiviral and is able to kick out the HPV virus without hesitation. Garlic had a major role in defeating small pox and the plague. This is amazing, wouldn't you agree?

The vaginal suppository protocol I used during the healing phase looked like this:
Always organic, eco-ly wildcrafted, and non-GMO.

Raw garlic 5 to 7 days　　　　　　Followed by douche 5 to 7 days

Take a day to rest, breathe, release, and place intention.

Herbal suppository 5 to 7 days　　Followed by douche 5 to 7 days
Astragalus root
Yellow dock root　　　　　　　　Distilled water and apple cider
Poke root　　　　　　　　　　　vinegar
Goldenseal
Turmeric
Echinacea

Tea tree oil
Cayenne pepper
Organic coconut oil
All ingredients were ground in
a coffee grinder and added to
OCO, placed in cylinders made
of aluminum foil, then refrigerated

Rest, and reassess whether an additional round of the suppository protocol is needed.

This formula is a mix from Dr. Schulze recommendation, I added additional herbs which felt wanted to be included.

When inserting the fine china suppository, place the herb side down, closest to the opening of fine china. I found when cleaning fine china the next day, it was much easier to retrieve all the plants from the fine china canal, and doing so during a salt and herbal bath was even easier.

"I come in too many flavors for one fucking spoon."

-Staceyann Chen

LOOSEN THE BOWELS

Simultaneously, treating the gastrointestinal tract, with emphasis on the colon, can assist and move out stuck and slow-moving toxins from the body and is of greatest importance. When we look at a disease like cancer, it is literally stuck emotions, stuck beliefs, and stuck body systems. I can say with integrity that my emotions, beliefs, and body systems had shut down prior to my diagnosis. When this happens, the disease is able to fester, replicate, and take over your well-being. Becoming unstuck has everything to do with increasing the frequency of bowel movements. For this job, I changed my diet, but also relied upon our herbal allies, as they toned and replenished me at every level of vibration, and assured the departure of stuck toxins.

I have a few favorites when choosing a bowel cleanser. The ingredients I seek are always made of our plant allies. Aloe vera was part of my smoothies, which the body fully consumes, ingests, and loves. There are many options to chose from for clearing toxins, but for this job I chose the Intestinal Movement Formula by Healthforce. To give you an idea of what a supplement made from our plant allies looks like, here are the ingredients:

Rhubarb root (turkey rhubarb is in the Essiac formula)
Peppermint leaf
Whole leaf aloe ferox
Nopal cactus or prickly pear
Ginger root
Thyme leaf
Oregano leaf
Chanca piedra whole herb
Enzymes - protease, amylase, cellulase, lipase, bromelan, papain

I would love to describe what each of these allies want to shout about:

Rhubarb root - (Rheum rhabarbarum)
This ally has been used to stimulate the production of red blood cells, used as a weight loss aid, assists with cardiovascular disease, aids in digestion, prevents Alzheimer's, improves bone health, prevents cancer, prevents macular degeneration, and is extremely high in vitamins and minerals.

Peppermint leaf - (Mentha piperita)
This ally has been used with IBS, gas, indigestion, colic, tuberculosis, hay fever, shingles, nausea, headaches, improves memory, treats radiation damage, herpes, assists in healing cavities and bad breath, and is antibacterial. Topically, it can be used for pain reduction, shingles, and herpes.

Whole Leaf leaf aloe ferox - (Aloe vera)
This very potent aloe vera plant has been used as a laxative, prevents cancer, heals skin disorders, promotes cellular growth, inhibits growth of microbes, is also harmful to certain types of bacteria and fungi, and is extremely high in vitamins and minerals.

Nopal cactus - (Opuntia)
Known as prickly pear has been used to reduce high cholesterol, obesity, hangovers, as a laxative, heals skin disorders, improves digestion, protects cardiovascular, boosts immune system, reduces insomnia, and is an anti-viral and anti-inflammatory.

Ginger root - (Zingiber officinale)
Ginger is enjoying its time of notoriety, and it's very well deserved. GR has been used to aid digestion, lower cholesterol, slow growth of cancer, ease nausea, decrease blood sugar, as an anti-spasmodic it aids in motion sickness or stomach aches. It's an anti-inflammatory,

aids menstruation, anti-viral, anti-fungal, anti-bacterial. Ginger is a warming circulatory herb, can be used both internally or externally, and is one of the top 30 herbs on the California School of Herbal Studies (CSHS).

Thyme leaf - (Thymus vulgaris)

Thyme has been used to boost the immune system, reduce anxiety or reduce the stress hormone, aids vision and slows the onset of macular degeneration, anti-fungal, high in potassium, therefore great for the heart, prevents strokes, heart attacks, and heart disease, highest anti-oxidant in the plant kingdom, is a warming and circulatory herb.

Oregano leaf - (Origanum vulgare)

Oregano has been used to balance the good / bad gut bacteria, digestive aid, ease bone and joint pain, boost the immune system, liver support and detoxification, anti-bacterial, antioxidant, anti-viral, and anti-spasmodic.

Chanca piedra whole herb - (Phyllanthus niruri)

This herb I have an affinity for, as I suffered from extreme kidney pain a few times within a year, and my acupuncturist believed the pain was due to a kidney stone(s) versus kidney infection. My chosen protocol was of course my herbal allies. I used the tincture Stone Breaker by Herb Pharm. I had a combo of arnica gel and pills, Stone Breaker, uva ursi, dandelion root, and lemon water, taken frequently over a period of a few days. My personal dosage exceeded the recommended dosage, because I am familiar with how my body responds to plant allies, but until you too are able to know your body, use the recommended dosage. After a few days, I passed the blockage, which showed up as heavy brown, sandy mucus in my stools. Gross. I have not had a reoccurrence. The nickname for the Chanca Piedra is "Stone Breaker" and our introduction to one another was pure magic. Stone Breaker has been used to support bladder, kidneys, gallbladder, and liver. Used to detoxify, strengthen, and heal liver from abuse of acetaminophen, alcohol, and other toxins. Can reduce high blood pressure and high blood sugar, boosts immune system, antibacterial, anti-inflammatory, antiviral - herpes, HPV, HIV, and eliminates stones to sand and prevents new stones from forming.

Enzymes

Enzymes are part of this supplement, but are not recommended for long-term use when taken in supplement form. Your body re-supplies enzymes by manufacturing them or by receiving them. They come naturally from whole grains (brown rice, millet, quinoa, barley, oats), beans, organic veggies, fruits, raw juicing, and fermented foods. When enzymes are unavailable for use or underproduced, your body begins to cut back from various bodily functions., i.e., hair may become dry, nails may crack, skin may become dry. The more critical the underproduction, the more difficult the liver's ability to handle the excretion of waste products. Fifty percent of all enzymes utilized by the body are used to digest food. When there are insufficient enzymes available, the body steals them from other organs.

Evidence in America of inadequate nutrition and enzyme production correlates with the high number of indigestion aids sold. Without enough enzymes, the average person will digest about 30-70% of what they eat. This exchange of energy will eventually cause exhaustion. Lack of live enzymes will not permit food to be thoroughly digested, therefore weakening our immune systems, creating inflammation within the gut and GI tract, and moving into degenerative diseases.

Taking enzymes as a supplement, long-term is similar to artificial hormones and melatonin. The body can decide to stop production when they are already within the system. For instance, a man on testosterone injections will inevitably show signs the body has stopped production of testosterone altogether when the scrotum shrinks into pea size scrotums. At this point, testosterone production says "Why show up if I am not needed?" The person has now created a bigger issue to deal with than before they began the hormone supplement. There is a wonderful tincture from WishGarden Herbs called *Male Mojo* for men looking for hormone balance without artificial hormones. (Male mojo is reviewed within the apothecary.) As with melatonin, again the body just decides "Why do I need to do the work in producing this amazing sleep hormone, when it's already here?" To reset the circadian rhythm, set aside time to feel the sun and moon's rays. It's completely free and absolutely works.

Enzymes should be used as a tool when deep healing is needed, not as a way of life. Find the diet that works for your body systems. Using bitters is a wonderful way to begin natural production of enzymes, and I always recommend bitters after any type of cleanse. By ending a cleanse with bitters (Wishgarden Herbs tincture - Bitters; Fenugreek, Oregon Grape root, Gentian root, Yarrow aerials, Orange peel, Hops strobiles) you are assuring balance and natural symmetry of all the body systems. Beautiful bitters can assist with subduing the pesky sweet tooth. Note, bitters can be used anytime you feel little off and are not limited to times of cleansing.

This concludes the Intestinal Movement Formula. Do you feel this supplement would have increased my vibrational frequency during the healing process? Yes, of course you do. Truly amazing allies, please take a bow.

"All disease begins in the gut."

-Hippocrates

"If you obey all the rules, you will miss all the fun."

-Katherine Hepburn

HERBAL ALLY CAPSULES:

We have met the fine china suppository and the bowel cleanser herbal allies. Next, I would like to introduce you to the rest of the tribe: the herbal ally capsules used to catapult my body systems to optimum vibrational frequency. These were taken every 1 to 3 hours to bring movement of blocked pathways, taken apart from one another. So basically I took these allies continuously throughout the days.

Additional Herbal Allies

Lifeshield by New Chapter Mushroom Complex
Echinacea & goldenseal
Astragalus
Vitex
Dandelion root
Probiotics

While some of these allies have already been introduced with the fine china suppository formula, we have a few newbies that truly deserve their day of appreciation.

Mushroom Complex
Vitex
Dandelion root
Probiotics

Mushroom Complex Lifeshield by New Chapter - This supplement is another example of a whole food, vibrational, intelligent supplement. Each mushroom is whole, with all constituents alive and ready to transmute their own job responsibilities into our being. The study of medicinal mushrooms dates back thousands of years.

The fungi family is part of Gaia's gifts to humanity and continues to blow my mind with their abilities to shift the mind/ body/ spirit into optimum health. I would like to introduce the medicinal mushrooms within the supplement: reishi, shitake, turkey tail, maitake, lion's mane, and chaga. I make it a point to bring these allies into my kitchen and sauté, bake or add them to soup and broths, assuring they are a constant part of my life.

Reishi has been known to boost immune response, bring vitality and strength, support adrenal function, alleviate chemotherapy side effects, i.e., nausea/ kidney damage, and protects DNA.

Shitake has been known to boost immune response, support liver, enhance mood, and is an anti-cancer that will eat cancer cells, and is anti-tumor. This ally is a favorite within the macrobiotic community.

Turkey tail has been known to boost immune response, can enhance effects of chemo and reduce side effects of radiation, relieves fatigue, anti-inflammatory and anti-cancer, and anti-tumor.

Maitake provides long-term immune enhancement, protects cells, fights infection, inhibits the spread of cancer, balances blood sugar, lowers cholesterol, and is an antioxidant, and anti-cancer.

Lion's mane has been used as a nervine, relieves anxiety and depression, strengthens immune system, enhances the digestion system, is anti-cancer, reduces cholesterol, heals ulcers, is an antioxidant, and assists with brain function: trauma, Parkinson's, Alzheimer's.

Chaga boosts the immune system, provides digestion support, anti-inflammatory, and is an anti-cancer agent - promotes apoptosis (natural progression of programmed cell death, but cancer cells do not go through this natural life cycle and become immortalized).

As you can see, these mushroom allies go deep within our anatomy. When we look at their ability to protect DNA upon replication, we bear witness to healing the most vital part of human anatomy. I find astragalus to be among our plant allies that encompass the same gift. Protecting our DNA upon replication is the most expressive gift of love from Gaia. Again, I will ask: "Do you think this supplement would raise my vibrational frequency or decrease it? I believe Gaia has done it again: raise, raise, raise me up, and I express deep gratitude and invite them all to take a bow. The next herbal allies which were apart of my healing phase, echinacea, goldenseal, astragalus and turmeric, have already been introduced with the vaginal suppository formula. These herbs were also taken in capsule form, and astragalus root and turmeric were also part of daily tea consumption and meal prep.

Vitex - (Vitex agnus-castus)

The next ally I would like to present is Vitex. Vitex and I have a history with it assisting me in finding hormonal balance, and it was used by my daughter when she first began her cycle. For years her cycle was sporadic and there was no way to know when or if she would have her cycle each month. We used Vitex to gently bring her body to balance and allow her cycles to find their rhythm. Vitex not only brought balance to fluctuating hormones, it softened pains associated with menses, and calmed her mood fluctuations, which was for my personal joy. That is amazing, wouldn't you say?

There is a connection to vaginal squamous cell malignancy and hormonal imbalance, and Vitex was my champion during the healing process. Herbal allies that balance the body's hormone levels are to be taken tonically (over a period of months). Vitex deserves its day in the spotlight, and here are some additional benefits our bodies receive from it.

Vitex has been used to relieve P.M.S. symptoms including irritability, mood swings, cramps, and breast tenderness, reduces uterine fibrosis, clears acne, treats endometriosis, balances estrogen and progesterone by increasing the luteinizing hormone (stimulates ovulation) and modulates prolactin which can increase lactation after birth, can prevent miscarriage (many are due to low progesterone, recommended into 3rd month of pregnancy), reduces menopause systems- minimizes hot flashes, stabilizes the menstrual cycle - great after stopping the birth control pill, induces ovulation, supports endocrine system, normalizes pituitary gland (the master gland for hormone production) and the hypothalamus.

Remember, this again is intelligent vibrational medicine. These allies know when or if the body is low on estrogen, and they will do their job and raise estrogen to a level which the body needs. If the body is high in estrogen, this ally will lower the hormone production level. To step into vibrational healing, there is a part of us which needs to surrender, get out of the spinning thoughts produced by fear or ego, connect with the deep knowing one can only find during meditation, and trust in the process. Breathe.

Vitex, please take your bow.

I would like to share with you a story regarding a recent hormonal disturbance within my own body. At the time of diagnosis, I was 45 years old. I am now 49 and ecstatic to share what has brought balance to me on all levels. Recently, my cycle began to arrive every two weeks. This was not painful, but at 49, I am beginning to shift out of baby-making times. I take Vitex, dong quai, and calcium/magnesium (algae and whole food source) monthly before the beginning of my cycle to assist the balance and bring harmony. I have not had any other disturbances, i,e., hot flashes, but having your menstrual cycle twice every month is a huge bummer, am I right? Again, I turned to Gaia to bring balance, and found a tincture by WishGarden Herbs called Wise Changes. Within the first month of taking this tincture, my cycle moved to every three weeks. By the second month, it moved to every 26 to 28 days, which is where I remain. Other benefits I received were truly restful sleep. Although I never had horrible nights' rest, I just felt rested. I also noticed my breasts looked amazing, toned, felt as if all the insides had firmed and softened at the same time, and little bumps which had come around each cycle, were also gone (I was also applying a creme called keeping abreast of it, by Simply Divine Botanicals.). My hair felt fuller around my face, which is where hair thins during hormonal disturbance. I felt blissful in many ways. Wise changes is reviewed at the end of the Apothecary.

We have reviewed the vaginal formula, the bowel movement formula, the mushroom complex formula, astragalus, turmeric, garlic, OCO, blended goldenseal & echinacea, and vitex. Dandelion is the remaining ally, and this herbal medicine was taken in tincture form and added to organic green tea daily, while dandelion greens were added to my salads and raw juices.

Dandelion - (Taraxacum)

Dandelion is known as a pesky weed, and the roots grow very deep into the soil, giving way to its extremely nutritive properties. Dandelion is among the top 30 herbs for CSHS, known as the best source for potassium. A diuretic, it restores vitality and is a liver tonic, has a cooling effect, detoxifies the liver, is a digestive aid, promotes bile production, increases bile flow, decongests the gallbladder, moves waste into the blood to be cleaned by the liver, relieves skin disorders, diabetes, acne, jaundice, cancer, anemia, maintains bone health, regulates blood pressure, lowers blood cholesterol, is a bitter, and a mild laxative.

This may be one of the oldest allies, and dates back 30 million years. Look around your home to notice which ally grows around you. These allies are Gaia giving a gift, and exactly what you need to help bring harmony into your life.

The last team member is a probiotic. A probiotic can be taken while on antibiotics, and is recommended to take a few hours after taking the antibiotic. Probiotics should be taken during the cold and flu season. Probiotics are the good bacteria, and can be consumed through fermented foods or supplements. These power-house allies support the immune system, assist with diarrhea, improve mental states and depression, reduce cholesterol and blood pressure, are anti-inflammatory, reduce skin allergies, aid with IBS, ulcerative colitis, Crohn's disease, and assist in weight loss. Foods high in probiotic activity are sauerkraut, miso, kimchi, kombucha, and pickled vegetables. Enjoy, and have fun.

"The doctor of the future will give no medicine, but will interest his patient in the care of the human frame, in diet and in the cause and prevention of disease."

-Thomas Jefferson

REVIEW

Always organic, non-GMO gives highest level of vibration.

First week garlic suppository, begin herbal capsules:

Raw organic garlic 5 to 7 days insert into fine china

Followed by douche 5 to 7 days Distilled water and apple cider vinegar

Herbal Ally Capsules
Mushroom complex
Astragalus
Vitex
Dandelion tincture
Turmeric
Goldenseal/Echinacea echinacea are short term allies taken for 2/3 weeks not to be taken tonically

Capsules should be taken tonically, over a few months

Take a day to rest every week, breathe, release, and place intention.

Second week herbal suppository, continue with herbal capsules:

Herbal suppository 5 to 7 days
Astragalus root
Yellow dock root

Poke root
Goldenseal
Turmeric

Followed by douche 5 to 7 days

Distilled water and apple cider vinegar

Echinacea
Tea tree oil
Cayenne pepper
Organic coconut oil
All ingredients were ground in
a coffee grinder and added to
OCO, placed in cylinders, sealed and refrigerated

Rest, and reassess whether an additional round of suppository protocol is needed.

"Above all, Be your own Hero."

-Rhea Iris Rivers

ADDITIONAL ALLIES - SOMETHING TO SHOUT ABOUT:

These allies are taken monthly before the beginning of my cycle. With each ally, I will describe their purpose as I have previously. I would love to go as deeply into each plant as I have with yellow dock and astragalus, but the purpose of the book is to introduce, raise vibrational frequency, and create curious researchers.

Dong quai and calcium/magnesium whole food supplements:

Dong quai - (Angelica sinensis)

I would like to introduce dong quai. I take this in capsule form and this ally has so much to shout about. DQ has been used for thousands of years, like most herbal allies, used with both men and women. It is known as a female ginseng but holds much value for men, such as: good for fertility in both men and women (by bringing balance to hormone levels), can raise the libido, treats premature ejaculation, used as a blood tonic or a blood cleanser as it removes toxins, blood thinner, high in biotin and folic acid and vitamin B12, reduces depression and mood swings, antispasmodic - reduces PMS pain and symptoms, balances estrogen levels, great for coming off birth control pill to normalize hormone production and regulate the cycle. Stops hot flashes. DQ can prevent pregnancy, stimulate the menstrual cycle, and release the lining of the uterus as well as a retained placenta. (The frequency and amount of dosage, gives this ally different job responsibilities) This ensures a supple, soft uterine wall and ease of pregnancy when one is ready for parenthood. DQ is not to be taken after the first day of the cycle has begun, as it brings on the rhythmic flow (blood), and once the flow has arrived, it is not necessary to bring on additional flow. I use this herb a few days before my cycle, unless there may be a chance of pregnancy (nature's birth control) then I use DQ after ovulation until the start of my cycle. Wow DQ!!!! Am I right? Such a champion for us. Please take a bow, DQ.

The calcium / magnesium (I take only whole food supplements, i.e., New Chapter or Tree of Life are both great, best source is from sea vegetables and algae.) I take this somewhat regularly, but always before and after my cycle. This supplement is also essential for children with ADHD/ADD, as using dairy for calcium will throw magnesium / calcium completely out of balance. Dairy is used to grow a calf into a very large cow within the first year of its life. It is simply too much for some human bodies, and more sensitive bodies can react with symptoms of ADHD/ADD, as my children did. Here are some of the reasons I use this supplement:

Plant-based, whole food magnesium has been used as an anti-inflammatory, to reduce cravings, assist preeclampsia symptoms, reduce osteoporosis, reduce foggy brain syndrome, assist with depression/anxiety, increase energy and vitality, reduce cramping of muscles, reduce headaches / migraines / mood swings, and to balance hormones, cycle and fertility. Calcium has been used to benefit and strengthen bones and skeletal development, used as a nervine and to assist nerve function, useful in blood clotting, the release of certain hormones, and to increase muscle control, including small muscle control truly needed by those with short attention spans and hyperactivity.

"I am willing to release that part of me that irritates me when I think of you."

-Doreen Virtue

Something to shout about, *Wise Changes*, a woman's tonic.

This tonic I used to bring balance to my cycle. I want to share with you all the other amazing benefits these allies bring into our lives. Wise Changes is a blended tincture of herbal allies and I believe these forgotten allies have been in hiding long enough. I would like to introduce Vitex berry (although in the vaginal suppository formula), motherwort aerials, black cohosh root, mugwort aerials, wild yam root, licorice root, burdock root, lady's mantle aerials, borage aerials, nettle leaf, and alfalfa leaf. When we increase or decrease the dosage of these allies it will change their actions. For hormone balancing it is recommend to take tonically (over a few months).

Currently, we have many books available for herbalists which give detailed actions to each of these allies. If you are seeking deeper knowledge please refer to The Holistic Herbal by David Hoffman, or The Complete Herbal Tutor, for further study.

Motherwort aerials - (Leonurus cardiaca)

Motherwort has been used for many, many moons and has been know to reduce risk of blood clotting, promote longevity and vitality, is a strengthening herb for blood and circulatory system, lowers cholesterol, can slow rapid heart rates and relieve stress on heart muscle, diuretic, reduce swelling, reduce gout, lower high blood pressure, balance hyper-thyroid. An antioxidant, it boosts the immune system, is anti-cancer, calms the central nervous system, is a nervine, reduces anxiety and depression, inhibits artery calcification, treats irregular heart rhythms, prepares the uterus for pregnancy, and can stimulate mild contractions (not recommended after pregnancy), brings balance to the menstrual cycle, relieves menstrual cramps, and is used with uterine fibroids, cysts, and endometriosis.

After researching many of our herbal allies I feel it is no wonder so much of our country suffers from many health issues. The further we detach ourselves from nature, the further out of whack our society is becoming. Motherwort, thank you for all your gifts.We remember you. Please take your bow.

Black cohosh - (Actaea racemes)

The next plant is black cohosh root. This ally is an at-risk plant and not to be wildcrafted. The California School of Herbal Studies has listed black cohosh among the top 30 plants to know, and has also asked that it be substituted with baneberry root when its pain relieving qualities are needed. This ally has been used by both women and men with benefits of reducing aches with the male reproductive system. It is a bitter, can be used to quiet a cough, nervine, supports the central nervous system, aids with depression, anxiety, mood swings, is useful with arthritis, rheumatoid arthritis, is an anti-spasmodic, anti-inflammatory, reduces heart disease and heart palpitation, headache, sleep disturbances, lowers HBP, improves immune system, is an antioxidant, reduces stomach acidity, indigestion, stomach cramps, can mimic hormonal activity, is useful in menopause for hot flashes, night sweats, and vaginal dryness.

What a beauty. Welcome back black cohosh. Please take your bow.

Mugwort aerials -(Artemisia vulgaris)

The next ally is mugwort aerials. This ally is also on the top 30 herbal allies from CSHS and has been used to balance irregular periods, induce late period, reduce cramping, treat PMS, stimulate the uterus - can cause miscarriage or release unwanted pregnancy, is a digestive aid, pain relieving, anti-spasmodic, anti-parasite, anti-candida, reduces insomnia and induces lucid dreaming. It can relax the mind while also keeping it alert. Reduces HBP, asthma, is a kidney and liver tonic, helps aid the absorption of nutrients, and is used with opium addicts to reduce addiction.

As I said previously, I am continually blown away at the level one can take their research into each of our herbal allies. I could get lost for days to weeks as a curious researcher, hungry for more knowledge. Mugwort, please take your bow and thank you.

Wild yam (Dioscorea villosa)

Wild yam is our next ally within Wise Changes. With so much to be excited about, this ally is our original birth control. Although we still do not understand for certain how wild yam affects our anatomy, it is believed that when used over two months at the right dosage, this ally will promote the growth of mucus around the woman's egg, thus not allowing the sperm to penetrate the egg (nature's birth control). Incredibly, when coupled with a condom and/or neem oil (which can kill sperm), we have ourselves something special. Additional uses for wild yam are to increase the libido in both men and women, anti-spasmodic, reduces abdominal and intestinal cramping, colic, nervine, balances central nervous system, anti-inflammatory, arthritis, rheumatoid arthritis, increases bile flow, reduces gallstones, moves liver congestion, balances endocrine system, balances progesterone and cortisol, lowers blood cholesterol levels, lowers HBP, is a diuretic that aids urinary system, and can increase or decrease fertility depending on the dosage and length of time taken.

I don't know about you, but I feel the need to curtsy for this ancient herbal ally. Truly here for mankind and womankind, wild yam is something special indeed.

Licorice root - (Glycyrrhiza glabra)

The next ally is licorice root, this ally is used within many herbal blends due to its delicious flavor, and it does extremely well when linked with other powerhouse allies. Licorice has been used as a digestive aid, lowers acidity, reduces ulcers, heartburn, soothes leaky gut, is an antibacterial, anti-inflammatory, antioxidant, antiviral, fights harmful organisms, helpful with dental health and gum disease, enhances immune system, promotes balance of yeast and fungus, respiratory aid expectorant, balances adrenal glands, increase vitality by balancing cortisol, anti-cancer, anti-depressant, prevents heart disease, antidepressant, aids menopause and reduces hot flashes. Licorice has been used for licorice candy, but the downfall is when used in candy, the sugar content decreases or completely eliminates every one of these benefits. That's right. Sad, but true.

Thank you licorice, please take your bow.

Burdock root - (Arctium lappa)

This next ally is used in the Essiac formula, and is a true friend to the human anatomy as well as our canine BFFs. Burdock root has a cooling effect on the body, and has been used as an antibacterial, anti-fungal, skin and blood cleanser, liver tonic/improves function, eliminates excess uric acid, highly nutritive, controls blood sugar level, reduces skin problems, anti-cancer, anti-tumor, boosts lymphatic system, reduces arthritis, cleanses and protects the spleen, and reduces enlarged spleen.

This plant is ancient, majestic, and here to aid humanity.

Lady's mantle aerial - (Alchemilla)

Lady's mantle aerial is also in the Wise Changes formula, and the gifts this ally encompasses are many. Here are some of the reasons it was chosen to be in the formula. It has been known to regulate the menstrual cycle, relieve menstrual cramps and PMS, reduce symptoms of menopause, useful with fibroids, endometriosis, polycystic ovaries, is an anti-inflammatory, antioxidant, antibacterial, antiviral (especially HPV), hormone regulator for fertility, strengthens the uterus, protects from miscarriage, promotes weight loss, hair tonic, helps with diabetes, gout, sleep disorders, enhances milk supply and flattens the belly, helps with colitis, diarrhea, and anti-influenza activity.

What a beauty, thank you lady's mantle

Borage aerial - (Borago officinalis)

Borage aerial is the next ally in the Wise Changes formula. Borage oil is becoming quite popular and here are some reasons why: borage has the highest GLA, is an anti-inflammatory, is anti-cancer, improves liver function, reduces anxiety and depression, helps with rheumatoid arthritis, seborrheic dermatitis, psoriasis, eczema, premature aging, Alzheimer's and memory disorders, supports the respiratory system: coughs, colds and flu, reduces fat accumulation, aids weight loss, reduces HBP, and increases male fertility.

Cheers to borage.

Nettle leaf - (Urtica dioica)

Nettle leaf is one of those plants one would want to be stranded on an island with, as it is extremely nutritive, is an antihistamine, anti-inflammatory, relieves allergies, is a diuretic, reduces uric acid, reduces gout, reduces incontinence while being a diuretic, is a kidney and adrenal tonic, assists with arthritis, RA, osteoporosis, is used through pregnancy, and is great for men - used for male pattern baldness and reduces an enlarged prostate.

Here, here, nettle leaf.

Alfalfa - (Medicago sativa)

Alfalfa is also a highly nutritive plant, and when sprouted, it tops the list of most nutritive sprouts. It is also used as an antioxidant, lowers HBP, treats ulcers, strengthens digestion, high in enzymes, brings healthy appetite, is a blood and liver detoxifier, promotes healthy bowel movements, lowers cholesterol, reduces atherosclerotic plaque, and nourishes the pituitary gland (master hormone factory).

Thank you, alfalfa.

This is the Wise Changes formulation. It is complete with all body systems being called for duty. It is said that herbalists and women from Asian countries (or countries that have not developed the American lifestyle) have little to no symptoms of menopause. I am excited to continue my journey through womanhood and experience what many other woman have experienced before me. I enjoy using my body as a petri dish to rediscover Gaia's ancient knowledge. It is clear why my irregular cycles linked up relatively quickly after reviewing these eleven allies. I hope you found herbal allies that called to you for usage or developed within yourself the curious researcher. As we use these allies to receive their gifts for humanity, keep in mind that we also receive every nutrient within the plant as well as their vibrational frequency. This is living vibrational medicine. It is truly magical.

"Don't gain the world and lose your soul, wisdom is better than silver or gold."

-Bob Marley

FOUR THIEVES OF MARSEILLES:

There appear to be over a dozen versions of this ancient story, taking place in medieval times of the 1300s to 1700s. Here is one version. A group of thieves living beyond the cities during the plague and black death epidemic in Europe were robbing from the sick and the nearly dead. These thieves were able to maintain their health regardless of being in close contact with the diseased. After their capture they agreed to release their secret of how they remained free from the deadly disease in exchange for freedom or leniency. Their magical juice dates back to time with Hippocrates. In 1937 their recipe hung in the Museum of Paris. It is thought to be the original copy of the recipe.

3 pints of white wine vinegar handful of wormwood, meadowsweet, wild marjoram, sage
50 clove
2 ounces campanula roots, angelica, rosemary, horehound
3 measures of camphor

Place the mixture in container for 15 days, strain, express then bottle.

Use by rubbing it on hands, ears, and temples from time to time and when approaching a plague victim.

The magical juice is believed to chase away fleas, and carriers of the plague. (We know from reading previous chapters, the ability to keep carriers of the plague away was not the only action of these herbal allies).

In Provence Italy this mixture is currently sold as "seven thieves vinegar".

The first time I heard this story I was in my Aromatherapy Course. The story transfers into essential oils of clove, cinnamon, rosemary and lemon. After the release of the recipe of the magical juice, the doctors began to wear duck bill face coverings and long robes. Within the duck bills the doctors inhaled dried herbs and essential oils. This was to ward off bacteria, fungus and viruses. The long robes worn by the doctors were also soaked in the magical juice, keeping them safe.

I found the correlation between the thieves living in the woods, still connected to Gaia and the ancient herbal ally knowledge fascinating. It seems the thieves stayed connected to nature, while the townspeople lived in bacteria-filled environments (before modern day sewage systems), devoid of this ancient healing knowledge. While the townspeople appear to be immersed in fear of herbal healing or said witchery the thieves seem to have all the answers to maintain health. During these ancient times the casting out of herbalists or said witches was a frequent occurrence. This allowed the banished herbalists to live away from the townspeople and within nature and stay connected to ancient wisdom. The towns people were then left ill-equipped to handle this epidemic without the use of natures forgotten healing herbal allies. I say to our plant kingdom once again, thank you.

"But ask the animals, and they will teach you, or the birds in the sky, and they will tell you; or speak to the earth, and it will teach you, or let the fish in the sea inform you. Which of all these does not know that the hand of the LORD has done this? In his hand is the life of every creature and the breath of all mankind." Job 12:7-10

CONSTITUTION - POTTENGER'S CATS:

This enlightening study was shown while attending one of my nutrition courses. It allowed me to view food and lifestyle on so many alternative levels and I truly enjoyed the film. The study took place from 1931-1942 and involved approximately 900 cats over a period of ten years, with three generations of cats studied. Note: During the 1930's GMO seeds or the use of growth hormones were not being used in our farming; therefore, the raw meat and raw dairy are considered somewhat organic. Here are the highlights from the study:

Meat study; control groups

One group of cats were fed 2/3 raw meat (organ meat, meat, bone), 1/2 raw milk, and cod-liver oil.

Second group of cats were fed 2/3 cooked meat (organ meat, meat, bone). 1/3 raw milk and cod-liver oil.

The cats fed the all-raw diet were healthy and full of vibrational zest for life, while the other group developed various health problems.

The 1ˢᵗ generation developed degenerative diseases and became lazy by the end of life. Second generation showed early onset of degenerative disease by mid-life and started to become uncoordinated with slow reactive response. Third generation showed very early onset of degenerative disease while some were born blind and weak with shorter life spans. Many of the third generations cats were unable to breed successfully. Those that were born did not survive six months. Kitten bones became soft and weak and they suffered from adverse personality changes. The males became submissive while the females became aggressive. There were noticeable parasitic infestations and vermin, while skin disruptions and allergies increased from 5% in normal cats to over 90% in 3ʳᵈ generation cats. These cats suffered from almost every degenerative human disease and died out by the end of the 4ᵗʰ generation, unable to breed.

Milk Study:

The cats were fed 2/3 milk and 1/3 meat. All groups were fed raw meat but the milk was different in each group: raw, pasteurized, evaporated, sweeten condensed, and vitamin D milk. The cats on the raw milk were the healthiest, while the other groups showed similar health problems to the meat study.

Let us revisit our constitution. Our constitution is the strength of our vibrational essence. Some people may be more prone to health crisis than the next person; this is due to the level of nourishment while in the womb. Regardless of constitution, by changing the variables i.e., stress or organic foods, we can move into stronger constitutions. Epigenetics has shown 1% of disease is due to genetics. This is what the study of the healing arts teaches, before the release of Epigenetics. Pottenger's cats relays a very clear connection to degenerative disease and food choices. When we look at our society and the current health crises and then examine the wombs of our moms-to-be, we can see correlations from weak bones, slow reaction time, skin disorders, bacteria invasions, adverse personality traits and the inability to conceive among many people within our communities.

During the viewing of this video what I found to be most interesting was at the completion of the study, once all the cats were released, the weeds, grass and other plants and insect life grew furiously in the raw food containments. But, when viewing the containments of cats with degenerative diseases their was little to no life growing from the soil, a ghost town. This leads me to ask, "how truly toxic are the droppings of humans who are riddled with ill-health? How is this affecting Gaia?" When revisiting my time with Rex, once I changed his food into part raw with home-made bone broths, I could see my lawn begin to grow beautifully without any dead spots. My lawn was vibrant and beautiful just like him.

"The greatness of a nation and its moral progress can be judged by the way its animals are treated."

-Gandhi

DOG MEAT:

This story begins with an evening at a friend's home. She had adopted an abused dog, a wolf-blended breed. This dog had previously snapped at my hand and bitten my finger. Also, this dog had attempted to bite two other people. This evening the dog had completed a long training session, over a few months with professionals in their field. I love animals and wanted to give this animal another chance, so I played ball with him, trying to bond, and gave him treats. This was the first time he was off leash. But when I turned my back on him, he attacked me from behind. He bit my golden round butt-rump first, and as I turned to face him he got ahold of my arm. I screamed, of course, and he released me, but continued his pursuit. Showing his razor sharp teeth and intense crazy eyes, he zeroed in on my throat, my jugular, hunting me as he growled deeply. I stepped backward into a corner. When I realized it was me or him, I began to move to the kitchen to grab a knife, yes, to stab him. He attacked me again and I grabbed a kitchen chair because the knifes were still too far away, and began using the chair as if I were in a lion's cage. I screamed at him like I've never known I was able, and lunged the chair at him to stop his attack. My advance broke his intense stare on my throat, and he then trotted away as if nothing had happened. I stood there with puncture wounds to my arm and finger, in a state of shock.

I do not feel every animal can be rehabilitated, but I believe we should try and then let go of them when the safety of our communities are at stake.

It turns out I received a maximum dosage of knowledge from this experience and felt my confidence soar as an herbalist. The protocol used for healing gave me even more confidence in the saying: nature has everything we need for wellness. The trick is we need to know which herbs and dosage, which is dependent on the depth of illness and can vary from person to person, depending upon one's constitution. I had another opportunity to become the petri dish and to learn first hand the power of our forgotten allies.

After the attack I soaked my finger and arm in warm salt water and essential oil of thyme and other allies, with alternated ice packs. The next morning my arm was sore but there was no sign of swelling. I began a regimen of goldenseal/echinacea, astragalus, fresh ginger, turmeric, and other teas. I believed I was going to get through this with little physical trauma, however, by the next day I felt horrible and a slight fever developed. My head and body began to ache with shooting pain at the top of my spine into my brain. I did not take any pain relievers, as I wanted to feel exactly what was happening within each of my body systems. My desire for more knowledge kept me from going to the emergency room as well as not wanting my friend to worry about the cost of a hospital visit. I also had the thought what if this bacteria has built up an immunity to antibiotics, then I would be worse off than staying on the path of discovery. (I do not recommend my choices, I am very in tune with my body and always enjoy opportunities for growth, but if it had been one of my children I would of had them in the emergency room right away.)

I brought additional allies into the treatment: Kick-ass biotic from Wishgarden Herbs taken every 1 to 3 hours. But by the evening the bacteria was winning the battle as I lay there feeling something that I've never experienced. From the puncture wound I felt a burning hot ball roll its way up my arm and into my left lymph node, igniting acute, intense pain and swelling. Within a few minutes my throat was on fire, and the pain moved to the right lymph node. My throat began to fill with mucus, as I suspected, this would be home base for the bacteria to breed, within their own biofilm. I was at a loss for what to do, was unsure of which ally I needed in the formula, and was having difficulties thinking straight due to the intense pain. It was 1am and thought if I'm alive by the morning I will go to the emergency room. It is then that I thought, why don't I practice what I preach and body scan, meditate, and ask divine for guidance? To become your own healer, you need only listen to your inner-guidance. Well, bingo.

As I looked within I asked, "What am I missing in my formula?" what I heard was that this bacteria attacks the blood and prevents the lymphatic system from doing its job. I needed additional blood cleansers and lymphatic herbs (these allies were in the blended tincture, but I needed a higher dose). I also needed to destroy the habitat it was breeding in: the mucus in my throat. Of course I thought, it made so much sense, and I thanked all that is divine for their assistance.

I brought in tinctures of burdock root, red root, and cleavers (these are the allies I had in my apothecary at 1am, thank god) while maintaining the other herbal allies. I was again amazed when the shooting pain from the top of my spine traveling into my brain began to subside within 15 to 20 minutes. I also gargled with warm Himalayan salt water, heavy on the salt, to destroy this invader's habitat, frequently. I was able to fall into a deep slumber, with little pain remaining, and in the morning I felt noticeably better. I woke and went into work, not totally on my A game but happy to be up and about.

I continued with the allies for another week to ensure the invaders' departure. With all respect to this bad-ass bacteria, it completely shut down my lymphatic system within forty-eight hours. Our lymph system is our anatomy's first line of defense, and when this system shuts down it is as if the castle wall has been removed, allowing for invaders from all directions to enter our domain. I consider this bacteria highly intelligent, vicious, and hungry for my soul. The battle was a struggle, but victory was mine. It is such a gift to know our plant allies. I am eternally grateful for all they have done for me and my family.

After the physical trauma had been released, I had emotional trauma to deal with. It came to my attention after speaking with a friend who happens to be a psychologist, that I was experiencing symptoms of PTSD, from the elevated heart rate to a spinning mind,

I felt the fight or flight response continually release. My eyes were in a state of panic, and my pupils appeared as black dots. During the attack, my daughter had arrived at the front door, and her knock is what turned my attention from the dog and allowed him to attack me from behind. When she heard my scream she yelled for me and wanted to enter the home. I told her, "Do not come in." I heard her attempt to open the door. Thank god it was locked. I play this mental image in my mind repeatedly: what if she'd entered? Could she have handled the attack? I would grow short of breath and begin feelings of panic, repeatedly, remembering the fear I had felt.

I've been through a lot in my life but never PTSD. It's amazing that much of the cure is found in meditation. I continued to refocus on the present moment, knowing my daughter was safe and I was safe, knowing that her safety was just a vision. As an avid meditator I could feel these assumptions enter my mind, but found myself overrun with emotions and unable to get ahold of myself. The reality of the vicious dog attack and the survival of an unsafe beast in my community rattled my core. I realized I could not shake this alone and needed additional help, and again I turned to Gaia. I looked to our forgotten allies, and trusted Wishgarden blended tinctures once again. The tinctures emotional ally and deep stress were consumed hourly, 3 to 5 times a day, and when in acute emotional stress I consumed them every 15 minutes. Wow, they really allowed me to get ahold of my emotions so I could begin the process of releasing what was not serving my best self. I could feel the slowing of the stress release pumping through my veins, instantly. These tinctures are complete magic without the risk of side-effects. I am forever on their team and am honored to known them.

I would like to highlight the amazing allies I used for healing:

Kick-ass Biotic (Wishgarden):
    Usnea Lichen - is an algea/fungus combination. It is anti-microbial, anti-bacterial, anti-fungal. It has the ability to heal wounds topically

and internally, heals staph infections, heals wounds, respiratory issues, urinary infections, sinus infections, vaginal infections, and provides allergy relief.

Bee propolis - known a bee glue, holds the hive together. It is useful in soothing eczema, psoriasis, is an anti-bacterial, anti-microbial, anti-inflammatory, immune boosting, destroys warts, cold sores, reduces allergies' histamine response, and fights cancer by causing cancer cells to die without harm to healthy cells (necrosis).

Myrrh gum - flea and tick repellant, pain relief for PMS or blood stagnation, anti-inflammatory, anti-fungal, anti-microbial, used against conjunctivitis, cold sores, and canker sores.

Goldenseal - refer to fine china suppository recipe

Baptisa root - Pain relieving, prevents cancer, boosts immune system, improves digestive system, used to treat ulcers, protect the respiratory system, is an anti-inflammatory, anti-bacterial, anti-oxidant, and can be mixed with poke root or cleaver for heavy lymphatic treatment (very powerful, use respectfully).

Red root - used topically for wound healing and sores of venereal disease, astringent, expectorant, sedative, heavy lymphatic support, digestion support, reduces bloating, indigestion and constipation, lung conditions, shortness of breath, and boosts the immune system.

Hops strobiles - Sedative to the central nervous system, treats anxiety, stress and insomnia, purifies the blood, treats impetigo, mange, leprosy, relieves congestion of the spleen, anti-viral, anti-microbial, anti-bacterial, and treats the urinary system.

Boneset aerials - This plant was named after its effective treatment of breakbone fever, a viral infection where one would have intense muscle pain, so much that they felt their bones would break. Aspirin replaced boneset. It is used to induce sweating for fevers and the flu, boost the immune system, and treat rheumatism, pneumonia, and gout.

Echinacea angustifolia root - This species was original to the Native Americans. Settlers brought echinacea purpurea from Europe, and there are varying opinions on which is more potent. I find Gaia will naturally produce the species which is needed most by humanity.

Enchinacea purpurea - refer to fine china suppository or supplements.

Emotional Ally (Wishgarden):
> *Motherswort* - refer to wise changes tincture.

Passionflower - Used for the central nervous system, relieves anxiety and panic attacks, supports normal sleep, is an anti-spasmodic, reduces muscle spasm, respiratory ailments, croup, whooping cough, asthma, epilepsy and severe digestive cramping, is restorative for emotional burnout, a natural ADHD alternative, calms internal chatter and allows better focus. It is used for drug addictions and withdrawal symptoms, opioid, and benzodiazepine addictions.

Milky oat tops - Treats the central nervous system, exhaustion, depression, anxiety and mental confusion.

Skullcap aerials - Part of the mint family. Relieves anxiety and pain, is an anti-inflammatory, soothes the central nervous system, reduces seizures, removes toxins, is an antioxidant, manages diabetes, lowers cholesterol, balances hormones, lowers risk of atherosclerosis, helps with weight loss, prevents cancer growth and tumor growth.

St. Johns wort aerials - Used for anxiety, depression, eczema, menopause, seasonal affective disorder, cold sores, and bedwetting.

Spikenard root - Antiseptic, purifies and detoxes, induces perspiration, fever reducer, used with gout, rheumatism, cough and respiratory issues, stimulates the immune system, reduces insomnia, depression, stress, anxiety, and chronic fatigue syndrome.

These are the heroes within emotional ally. Please take your bow. This tincture is a wonderful symptom-reliever. I was able to feel a shift after the first dose, which allowed me to rest and assimilate and begin to release the trauma. Thank you emotional ally.

Deep Stress (Wishgarden):

Nettles - refer to wise changes

Milky oat tops - refer to emotional ally

Borage - refer to wise changes

Skullcap - refer to emotional ally

Parsley leaf - Highly nutritive with vitamins and antioxidants. Pain relieving, fights cancer, halts tumor growth, prevents cancer growth, controls diabetes, treats rheumatoid arthritis, prevents osteoporosis, is an anti-inflammatory, assists digestion, treats cramps, indigestion, edema, nausea, strengthens the immune system, is a kidney cleanse, helps with weight loss, is collagen boosting, antibacterial, anti-fungal, boosts cardiovascular health, balances hormones, and promotes eye health.

Thyme leaf - Lowers blood pressure, cholesterol, is a cough remedy, boosts the immune system, is an antifungal, antibacterial, antiviral, antiseptic, has an uplifting effect on mood, and is highly nutritive.

Motherswort - refer to wise changes

Codonopsis root - Boosts the immune system, mental clarity and memory, helps the body handle stress, minimizes diabetes, supports liver and spleen, is a blood tonic and can increase red blood cells, minimizes adrenaline in fight or flight response, reduces fatigue, high blood pressure, headaches, and is a digestive tonic.

Holy basil aerials - Treasured in India, and known at Tulsi. Treats respiratory discomforts, fever, asthma, relieves congestion, heart disease and stress. Use the leaves in water before drinking to clear bacteria and fungus. The aroma can keep bacteria and viral infection away, is an anti-oxidant, reduces cholesterol, helps with dental care, prevents kidney stones, clears acne, relieves headaches, prevents premature aging, boosts immune system, inhibits growth of HIV and cancer cells, helps with eye care and skin care, and is an anti-parasitic.

Bladderwack frond - Is a sea vegetable, highly nutritive, improves metabolism by bringing balance to the thyroid, treats obesity, lowers risk of cancer, anti-inflammatory, and boosts circulation.

Peppermint leaf - Used to remineralize teeth, digestive aid, treats IBS, helps with weight loss, is a fever reducer, reduces nausea, treats motion sickness, gas, heartburn, nervine and improves circulation, is anti-cancer, improves liver function, and enhances memory.

Eleuthero root - also known as Siberian ginseng - boosts the immune system, boosts metabolism, increases circulation, nervine, reduces fatigue, increases blood to the brain, improves cognition and memory, relieves stress, slows or stops the advancement of Alzheimer's, is an anti-inflammatory, lowers high blood pressure, reduces cholesterol, controls diabetes, and improves respiratory health.

This completes the forgotten heroes within the magical tincture deep stress, from Wishgarden herbs. This tincture can be taken tonically, and can be taken acutely. Deep stress helps nourish over-stressed adrenals and brings comfort to the fight or flight response. This is another true ally for humanity.

Additional tinctures:

Cleavers, burdock, and red root are the additional tinctured allies brought in to the formula, to assist with blood cleaning and removal of lymphatic debris.

Cleavers (Galium aparine) - Used for its affinity for the lymphatic system, flushes lymph and kidneys, heals swollen glands, is a diuretic, cleans and purifies the blood, is an astringent and antiseptic, heals wounds, and prevents and clears urinary stones.

Red root (Ceanothus americanus) - refer to kick-ass biotic

Burdock root - refer to wise changes

Through this experience I have gained a tremendous amount of gratitude and knowledge. I have gained an entirely new point of view for our human heroes within our military and local support. I realize being attacked by a dog is minimal when looking at the ungodly amount of stress a solider or police officer may endure. I feel very grateful to these men and women for truly putting their lives on the line for humanity and realize the difficulties in dealing with PTSD.

"If you don't like the road you're walking, start paving another one."

-Dolly Parton

MALE MOJO:

This wonderful ally is a blended tincture (by Wishgarden). The master herbalist who designed this beauty is truly a plant intuitive. I have found that as men age, they too go through their version of menopause, and many of my male clients have enjoyed this tincture. When using our plant allies to balance hormone production, we open ourselves to vibrational uplifting energies to occupy our domain and allow for the balance of all hormones. As we age, our hormones are supposed to change. This shift allows for us to view life in new perspectives and hopefully on a deeper and more fulfilling level, while releasing past experiences rather than trying to continuously recreate them. I feel that we have been sold the idea: it's not okay to age, or to allow our hormones to shift. When we review the state within our communities and the link to hormonal disruptors, we can now see the connection to food, thoughts, stress, and basic lifestyle and how they effect our well-being. These forgotten allies use their plant intelligence to determine which hormone may need a higher level of production or which hormone may have been over-produced. This plant intelligence is useful to bring balance as these allies also know when enough is enough, and will reduce production, as needed.

When we change our diet and lifestyle we are able to reduce our degenerative diseases; this includes those of our reproductive system. A big part of these forgotten allies address the failing male prostate, as the prostate is seeking attention and needs additional nourishment as it ages. Although these allies work deeply within our anatomy, a change of lifestyle is recommended when one begins to experience loss of circulation within the genital area (men and women). This is just another opportunity to tune into your self and find what is no longer nurturing your best self. The body we develop after forty is not in any way shape or form the body we had in our twenties, and should be honored as such. The allies within this hero's delight are:

saw palmetto fruit, damiana leaf, Jamaican sarsaparilla root, burdock root, Oregon grape root, dandelion root, and yellow dock root.

The review of each forgotten ally:
   Saw palmetto fruit - The fruit can be eaten in its natural form or made into medicine. Useful for balancing hormones (men & women), treats male-female pattern baldness, treats impotence, increases performance and balances libido (men & women), prevents prostate cancer and heals inflamed prostate. Known to reduce kidney disorders, strengthens urinary disorders, can increase muscle mass, has an affinity for balancing testosterone. Testosterone is responsible for muscle mass increase, and also boosts the immune system.
   Damiana Leaf - Balances hormones (men and women), controls hot flashes, brings passion to one's life, relieves stress and anxiety, opens circulation in the genitals (men and women), treats erectile dysfunction, antidepressant, soothes the digestive system and removes toxins from the GI tract.
   Jamaican Sarsaparilla root - Introduced as a soft-drink long ago. Balances hormone production (men and women), treats male-female pattern baldness, hot flashes, anti-oxidant, prevents cancer, anti-inflammatory, treats pain of gout and arthritis, increases sex drive, circulatory herb, soothes PMS, used for infertility, nervine, psoriasis, acne, rashes, syphilis, is an antibacterial, boosts the immune system, aids in weight loss, appetite suppressant, skin care, detoxifies and purifies the blood, diuretic.
   Burdock root - refer to wise changes
   Oregon grape root - Used in place of endangered goldenseal, as they have similar properties. Anti-inflammatory, soothes the digestive system and GI tract, antibacterial, antioxidant, stimulates bile, moves stuck toxins from the liver, balances insulin, useful as a laxative, works against parasites and worms, useful with endometriosis, balances estrogen, psoriasis and sinus ailments.
   Dandelion root - refer to oral supplements
   Yellowdock root - refer to vaginal suppository

These wonderful forgotten allies are all part of allowing our bodies to find the perfect amount of hormone regulation, naturally and successfully. When we use a blended tincture the amount of each herbal ally is determined by the master herbalist.

Thank you Male Mojo.

"The best and most beautiful things in the world cannot be seen or even touched, they must be felt with the heart."

- Helen Keller

HOW TO SOAK:

Use raw grains, seeds, or legumes that have not been roasted, blanched, or prepared in any way.

Place them in a bowl covered with several inches of filtered water, and cover with a kitchen towel. For beans, add a carrot or potato to soak up gases within the beans. Let them sit for the desired length of time.

If soaking more than 12 hours, rinse the grains, nuts, seeds, or beans every 12 hours and change the water.

Do this every 12 hours for up to 48 hours with legumes. You'll notice how much they've expanded as they soak up water, which is a good thing. Rinse and cook.

After cooking, they will keep in the refrigerator. Use within the next week, adding to stir-fries, green salads, or soups… easy peasy.

HOW TO SPROUT:

To sprout seeds, nuts, and grains:
Soak and leave in the strainer, or in a shallow dish, somewhere they will be exposed to air.

Keep them slightly damp, but do not cover them in water completely. Use only 1-2 tablespoons of water.

Leave them out until the desired length of sprout is obtained. The length of time will vary depending on the kind of seed you're sprouting.

Sprouts will vary from 1/8 inch to 2 inches long. When ready, drain, rinse the sprouts well, and store in a jar or container.

Keep refrigerated for up to 7 days, rinsing daily in a fresh bowl to prevent harmful bacteria from growing. My favorite is radish sprouts: they really pack a pop.

Soaking and Sprouting Guide:

NUTS

Almonds - 2-12 hours for soaking, 2-3 days to sprout if truly raw
Walnuts - 4 hours for soaking, do no sprout
Brazil Nuts - 3 hours for soaking, no not sprout
Cashews - 2-3 hours for soaking, do not sprout
Hazelnuts - 8 hours for soaking, do not sprout
Macadamias - 2 hours for soaking, do not sprout
Pecans - 6 hours for soaking, do not sprout
Pistachios - 8 hours for soaking, do not sprout

BEANS & LEGUMES

Chickpeas - 8-12 hours for soaking, 2-3 days for sprouting
Lentils - 8 hours for soaking, 2-3 days for sprouting

Adzuki Beans - 8 hours for soaking, 2-3 days for sprouting
Black Beans - 8-12 hours for soaking, 3 days for sprouting
White Beans - 8 hours for soaking, 2-3 days for sprouting
Mung Beans - 24 hours for soaking, 2-5 days for sprouting
Kidney Beans - 8-12 hours for soaking, 5-7 days for sprouting
Navy Beans - 9-12 hours for soaking, 2-3 days for sprouting
Peas - 9-12 hours for soaking, 2-3 days for sprouting
Pinto - 8-12 hours for soaking, 2-3 days for sprouting

GRAINS

Buckwheat – 30 min-6 hours for soaking, 2-3 days for sprouting
Amaranth Grains - 8 hours for soaking, 1-3 days for sprouting
Kamut - 7 hours for soaking, 2-3 days for sprouting
Millet - 8 hours for soaking, 2-3 days for sprouting
Oat Groats - 6 hours for soaking, 2-3 days for sprouting
Quinoa - 4 hours for soaking, 1-3 days for sprouting
Wheat Berries - 7 hours for soaking, 3-4 days for sprouting
Wild rice - 9 hours for soaking, 3-5 days to sprouting
Black rice - 9 hours for soaking, 3-5 days for sprouting
Brown rice - 9 hours for soaking, 3-5 days for sprouting

SEEDS

Radish seeds - 8-12 hours for soaking, 3-4 days for sprouting
Alfalfa Seeds - 12 hours for soaking, 3-5 days for sprouting
Pumpkin Seeds - 8 hours for soaking, 1-2 days for sprouting
Sesame Seeds - 8 hours for soaking, 1-2 days sprouting
Sunflower Seeds - 8 hours for soaking, 2-3 days for sprouting
Chia Seeds - 2-4 hours for soaking, do not sprout
Flax seeds - 2-4 hours for soaking, do not sprout
Hemp seeds - 2-4 hours for soaking, do not sprout

"Political parties and World religions have yet to bring change for the World's needs, repeatedly. We the people are the change the World needs, by way of connecting through compassionate acts and conscious consuming."

-Rhea Iris Rivers

Printed in the United States
By Bookmasters